CW00802025

Practice Nursing

Clinical Guidelines and Procedures in Practice

THERESA LOWRY-LEHNEN

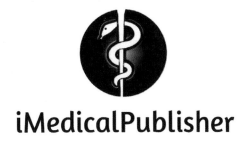

iMedicalPublisher

First edition: 2018

Art Director: Susana Robles_susan.art.dir@gmail.com

Edited version: iMedical Publisher
                   info@iMedicalPublisher.com
                   http://iMedicalPublisher.com

ISBN: 978-1-9993485-0-2

© All rights reserved. No part of this publication may be reproduced or transmitted in any form and by any electronic means, photocopying, recording and others without prior written permission of the authors and publishers.

Whether you are a nurse about to embark on a lifelong career or one who is already established in practice, this evidence based concise practical book serves as both a guide and a helping hand to provide the theory and principle, practical knowledge and confidence for all nurses. It is a must have for all practice nurses, both new and experienced to ensure we work towards best practice and ensure the highest standard of care for all our patients.

Dr. Maitiú Ó Tuathail

President NAGP (Ireland) 2018

Foreword

Practice Nurses play an important and pivotal role in healthcare providing a range of interventions and services to patients in General Practice and Primary Care settings.

While most Practice Nurses work in GP surgeries and doctor led clinics, others are working as autonomous practitioners in community practices and nurse led centres, such as Walk - in Centres, Student Health Centres, Occupational Health, Health Screening and Information Services, Community Intervention Team and Out Of Hours GP Clinical and Triage Nursing Services.

Practice Nurses are presented with an ever increasing range of conditions and patient needs as the role is constantly changing and evolving. The extended roles and range of clinical skills which may be provided by a Practice Nurse depend on the needs of the patient and the qualifications, skills, competencies and scope of practice of each individual Practice Nurse (NMBI 2015). Practice Nurses, therefore, have a responsibility to ensure that they are suitably qualified, skilled and competent in carrying out each clinical procedure and intervention that they undertake.

Practice Nursing: Clinical Guidelines and Procedures in Practice provides a comprehensive overview and a step by step guide for nurses carrying out a range of clinical procedures in General Practice and Primary Care settings. National clinical directives, policies, guidelines and documents are regularly updated and should always be consulted. This manual, written by a Practice Nurse, is based on current local and national guidelines. It is intended as a quick guide reference to clinical procedures commonly carried out in Irish health care settings, but main government publications, guidelines and updates should always be referred to.

Author

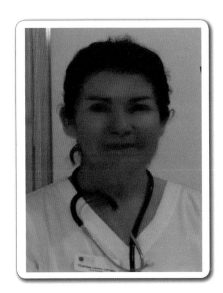

Theresa Lowry-Lehnen, RGN is qualified as a practitioner in General Practice Nursing and a Teacher of Science. She has a PhD, and has published a number of books and medical journal articles. Theresa is a graduate of MMUH, The Open University, NUIM, St. Mary's Teacher Training University College, London, The University of Surrey, and is a registered Teacher with the Teaching Council of Ireland. She has over 30 years' experience in clinical nursing practice, combining her practice with 14 years in educational, teaching and lecturing roles. Theresa was short-listed for the 'Practice Nurse of the Year' Award 2018, at the GP National Awards in Ireland. She is currently employed as an Associate Lecturer and the full-time Practice Nurse at the Medical Centre, Institute of Technology Carlow, Ireland.

RGN, Post Graduate Coronary Care, Dip.Counselling, BSc (Hon's) Specialist Practitioner in General Practice Nursing, MSc Nursing, PGCE (QTS) Science, H.Dip.Ed, MEd, PhD
Orcid ID: https://orcid.org/0000-0002-4889-4133

Table of Contents

1. Hand Hygiene Techniques

1. Guidelines for hand hygiene in Irish healthcare settings

Figure 1: Hand Wash Technique with Soap and Water.

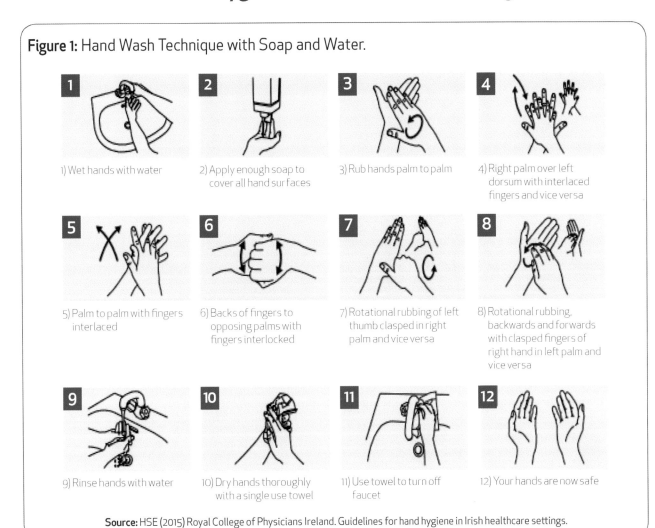

1) Wet hands with water

2) Apply enough soap to cover all hand surfaces

3) Rub hands palm to palm

4) Right palm over left dorsum with interlaced fingers and vice versa

5) Palm to palm with fingers interlaced

6) Backs of fingers to opposing palms with fingers interlocked

7) Rotational rubbing of left thumb clasped in right palm and vice versa

8) Rotational rubbing, backwards and forwards with clasped fingers of right hand in left palm and vice versa

9) Rinse hands with water

10) Dry hands thoroughly with a single use towel

11) Use towel to turn off faucet

12) Your hands are now safe

Source: HSE (2015) Royal College of Physicians Ireland. Guidelines for hand hygiene in Irish healthcare settings.

2. Guidelines for hand hygiene in Irish healthcare settings

Alcohol Hand Rub Technique

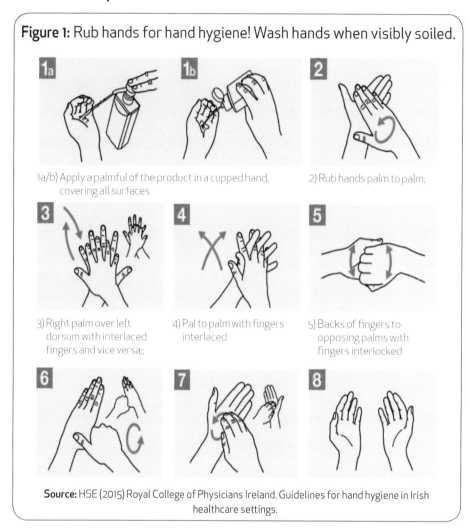

Figure 1: Rub hands for hand hygiene! Wash hands when visibly soiled.

1a/b) Apply a palmful of the product in a cupped hand, covering all surfaces

2) Rub hands palm to palm;

3) Right palm over left dorsum with interlaced fingers and vice versa;;

4) Pal to palm with fingers interlaced

5) Backs of fingers to opposing palms with fingers interlocked

Source: HSE (2015) Royal College of Physicians Ireland. Guidelines for hand hygiene in Irish healthcare settings.

3. Indications for hand hygiene

Clean hands according to the WHO '5 moments for hand hygiene':

1. Immediately before each episode of direct patient contact or care
2. Immediately before a clean/aseptic procedure
3. Immediately after contact with body fluids or excretions, mucous membranes, non - intact skin or wound dressings
4. Immediately after each episode of direct patient contact or care
5. Immediately after contact with objects and equipment in the immediate patient environment

4. Other indications for hand hygiene

Hands should also be cleaned:

- When visibly dirty, or soiled with blood or other body fluids
- After using the toilet
- Before preparing medication
- Before preparing food
- Before putting on gloves
- Immediately after removing gloves

5. Hand hygiene and glove use

The use of gloves does not replace the need for hand hygiene When using gloves, clean hands:

- before putting on gloves
- immediately after removal of gloves

6. When delivering clinical care

- Bare the wrists (e.g., short sleeved top or rolled up sleeves)
- Remove all wrist jewellery, including wristwatch
- Remove all hand jewellery (a single plain band may be worn)
- Keep fingernails short (tips less than 0.5cm)
- Do not wear false nails or nail enhancements (e.g., gel nails)
- Do not wear nail varnish
- Cover cuts and abrasions with a waterproof dressing

7. Which hand hygiene product to use

Use an alcohol hand rub for hand hygiene, except in the following situations when hands must be washed with soap and water:

- When hands are visibly soiled
- When caring for patients known or suspected to have Clostridium difficile infection

Alcohol hand rub used in healthcare settings should conform to the national specification for alcohol - based hand hygiene products

8. Hand hygiene technique

8.1 Alcohol hand rub

- Do not use alcohol hand rub on visibly soiled hands
- Follow the manufacturer's instructions for application times
- Apply sufficient volume of hand rub solution to cover hands and wrists
- The hand rub solution must come into contact with all surfaces of the hands and wrists
- Rub hands together vigorously until the solution has evaporated and hands are dry

8.2 Hand washing with soap and water

- Wet hands under running water. Avoid using hot water
- Apply sufficient amount of liquid or foam soap to cover all surfaces of the hands and wrists
- The soap solution must come into contact with all surfaces of the hands and wrists
- Rub hands together vigorously for a minimum of 15 seconds
- Rinse hands thoroughly
- Do not use clean hands to turn off taps
- If taps are not hands - free, use paper towel to turn off tap
- Dry hands thoroughly with disposable paper towels
- Discard towel into hands - free non - risk waste bin

8.3 Surgical hand preparation (may also be referred to as surgical hand hygiene)

- Surgical hand preparation should be performed using either an antimicrobial soap or an alcohol - based hand rub with persistent antimicrobial activity (surgical hand rub) prior to donning sterile gloves when performing surgical procedures
- Do not sequentially combine surgical hand preparation with antimicrobial soap and a surgical hand rub
- Remove all rings, wrist watch and bracelets
- Keep fingernails short (less than 0.5cm)
- Do not wear false nails or nail enhancements (e.g., gel nails)
- Do not wear nail varnish

- If hands are visibly soiled, wash with soap and warm water prior to surgical hand preparation
- Remove debris from underneath nails using a nail cleaner

8.4 Surgical hand preparation with antimicrobial soap

- When performing a surgical hand preparation with antimicrobial soap, scrub hands and forearms for the length of time recommended by the manufacturer, usually 2 - 5 minutes. Longer scrub times (e.g., 10 minutes) are not necessary
- Pay special attention to nails, subungual areas, between fingers and between thumb and index finger
- The direction of the washing procedure is from the hands to the elbows, without returning to the cleaned hands. Soap should be rinsed in the same manner
- Brushes should not be used
- Dry hands and forearms with a sterile towel, from the hands to the elbows
- Hands and forearms should be completely dry prior to donning gloves

8.4 Surgical hand rub with an alcohol - based hand rub with persistent antimicrobial activity

- When performing a surgical hand rub with an alcohol - based hand rub with persistent antimicrobial activity, follow the manufacturer's instructions for application times
- Hands and forearms should be dry before alcohol hand rub is applied
- Use sufficient product to keep hands and forearms wet with the hand rub throughout the surgical hand rub procedure
- After the surgical hand rub, allow the hands and forearms to dry completely prior to donning gloves

8.5 Prevention of skin damage

- Educate staff about the potentially damaging effects of hand hygiene products and of practices to reduce the risk of skin damage
- Use an emollient hand cream frequently
- Avoid using hot water for hand washing
- Avoid using soap and alcohol hand rub at the same time
- After hand washing, dry hands thoroughly with a patting motion rather than rubbing
- Avoid donning gloves while hands are wet

- Avoid prolonged and inappropriate use of gloves
- Consult the occupational health team or a general practitioner if skin irritation occurs from use of hand hygiene products in the healthcare setting
- Provide alternative hand hygiene products for healthcare workers with confirmed allergies or adverse reactions to standard products used in the healthcare setting

9. Hand hygiene facilities Alcohol hand rub

- Alcohol hand rub should be made available at the point of care in all healthcare facilities
- A risk assessment should be performed to ensure that there is no risk of accidental or intentional ingestion of alcohol hand rub at the point of care by the individual patient
- Alcohol hand rub used in healthcare settings should conform to the national specification for alcohol-based hand hygiene products
- Disposable single use alcohol hand rub cartridges or containers should be used

9.1 Hand washing facilities (Primary care)

- Clinical hand wash sinks should be dedicated for hand washing only and labelled accordingly
- Clinical hand wash sinks should conform to HBN 00-10 Part C Sanitary Assemblies
- Clinical hand wash sinks should be accessible and should not be situated behind curtain rails
- Clinical hand wash sinks should be located so that they are convenient for use
- Liquid or foam soap, disposable paper towels and warm water should be provided
- Hand driers should not be used in clinical areas
- Disposable single use soap cartridges or containers should be used
- Taps should be hands-free
- Where clinical procedures or examination of patients is undertaken in primary care and out-patient settings, a clinical hand wash sink should be provided where the procedure or examination is carried out

9.2 Emollient hand creams

- Emollient hand creams which are compatible with the hand hygiene products in use should be available in all clinical care areas
- Emollient hand creams should be provided in a wall mounted or pump dispenser. Disposable single use cartridges or containers should be used

9.3 Audit of hand hygiene

- Regular audits of hand hygiene (the nature of which should be determined locally) with feedback should take place in all healthcare settings, and should be linked to an improvement programme
- Hand hygiene audits should form part of a broader programme of surveillance and audit
- Audits should be performed in a standardised manner so that results can be compared over time
- Results should be reported to senior management, clinicians and the infection prevention and control committee (where present)

2. Summary of High - Quality CPR Components for BLS Providers

Component	Adults and Adolescents	Children Age 1 Year to Puberty	Infants Age Less Than 1 Year, Excluding Newborns
Scene safety	Make sure the environment is safe for rescuers and victim		
Recognition of cardiac arrest Activities	Check for responsiveness No breathing or only gasping (ie.no normal breathing) No definite pulse felt within 10 seconds (Breathing and pulse check can be performed simultaneously in less than 10 seconds)		
Activation of emergency response system	Alone with no mobile phone, leave the victim to activate the emergency response system and get the AED before beginning CPR. Otherwise, send someone and begin CPR immediately; use the AED as soon as it is available	Witnessed collapse Follow steps for adults and adolescents Unwitnessed collapse Give 2 minutes of CPR Leave the victim to activate the emergency response system and get the AED. Return to the child or infant and resume CPR; use the AED as soon as available	
Compression - ventilation ratio without advanced airway	1 or 2 rescuers 30:2	1 rescuer 30:2 2 or more rescuers 15:2	
Compression - ventilation ratio with advanced airway	Continuous compressions at a rate of 100 - 120/min Give 1 breath every 6 seconds (10 breaths/min)		
Compression rate	100 - 120/min		
Compression depth	At least 2 inches (5 cm)*	At least one third AP diameter of chest About 2 inches (5 cm)	At least one third AP diameter of chest About 1½ inches (4 cm)
Hand placement	2 hands on the lower half of the breastbone (sternum)	2 hands or 1 hand (optional for very small child) on the lower half of the breastbone (sternum)	1 rescuer 2 fingers in the center of the chest, just below the nipple line 2 or more rescuers 2 thumb–encircling hands in the center of the chest, just below the nipple line
Chest recoil	Allow full recoil of chest after each compression; do not lean on the chest after each compression		
Minimizing interruptions	Limit interruptions in chest compressions to less than 10 seconds		

*: Compression depth should be no more than 2.4 inches (6 cm). **Abbreviations:** AED, automated external defibrillator; AP, anteroposterior; CPR, cardiopulmonary resuscitation.
Source: Highlights of the 2015 American Heart Association, guidelines update for CPR an ECC.

3. BLS Healthcare Provider Adult Cardiac Arrest Algorithm- 2015 Update

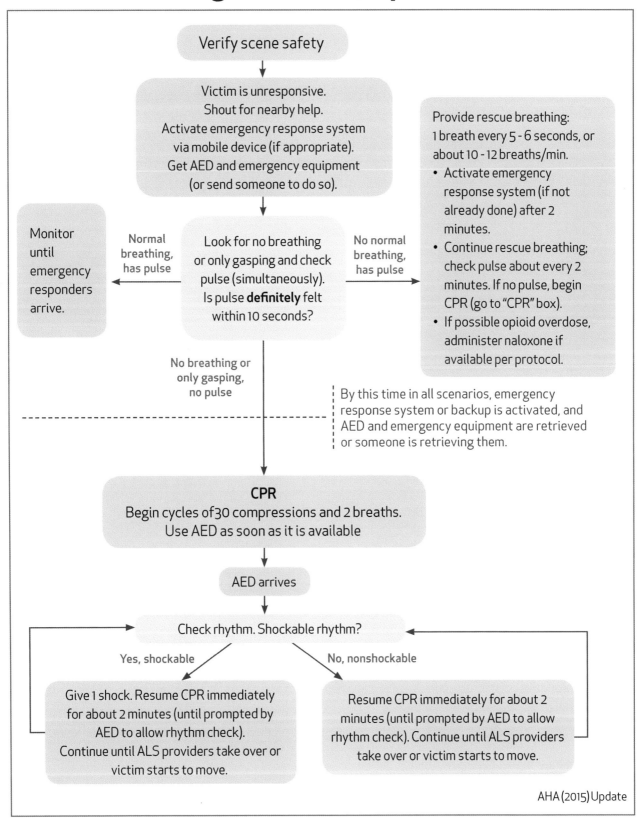

Verify scene safety

Victim is unresponsive.
Shout for nearby help.
Activate emergency response system
via mobile device (if appropriate).
Get AED and emergency equipment
(or send someone to do so).

Provide rescue breathing:
1 breath every 5 - 6 seconds, or
about 10 - 12 breaths/min.
- Activate emergency response system (if not already done) after 2 minutes.
- Continue rescue breathing; check pulse about every 2 minutes. If no pulse, begin CPR (go to "CPR" box).
- If possible opioid overdose, administer naloxone if available per protocol.

Monitor until emergency responders arrive.

Normal breathing, has pulse

Look for no breathing
or only gasping and check
pulse (simultaneously).
Is pulse **definitely** felt
within 10 seconds?

No normal breathing, has pulse

No breathing or only gasping, no pulse

By this time in all scenarios, emergency response system or backup is activated, and AED and emergency equipment are retrieved or someone is retrieving them.

CPR
Begin cycles of 30 compressions and 2 breaths.
Use AED as soon as it is available

AED arrives

Check rhythm. Shockable rhythm?

Yes, shockable

No, nonshockable

Give 1 shock. Resume CPR immediately
for about 2 minutes (until prompted by
AED to allow rhythm check).
Continue until ALS providers take over or
victim starts to move.

Resume CPR immediately for about 2
minutes (until prompted by AED to allow
rhythm check). Continue until ALS providers
take over or victim starts to move.

AHA (2015) Update

4. BLS Healthcare Provider Paediatric Cardiac Arrest Algorithm (Single Rescuer)

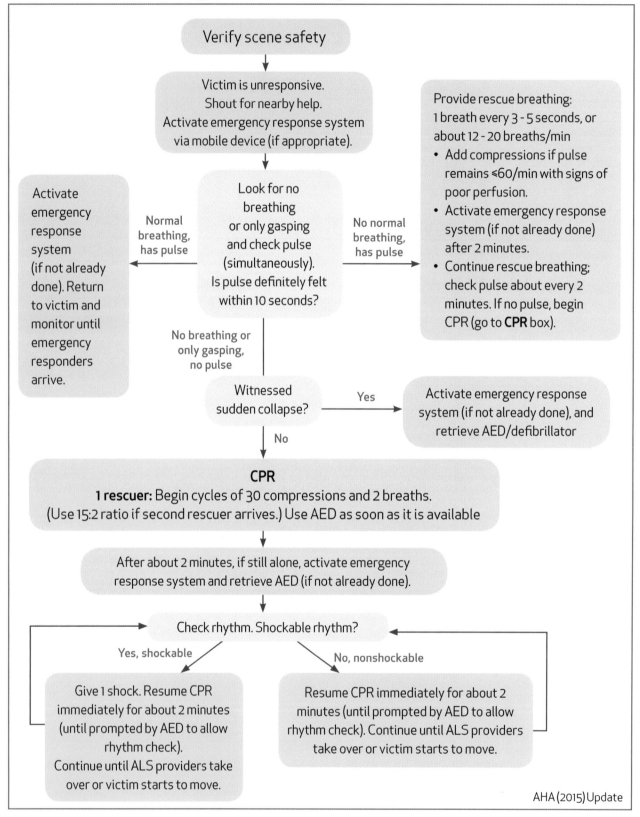

Verify scene safety

Victim is unresponsive.
Shout for nearby help.
Activate emergency response system
via mobile device (if appropriate).

Look for no
breathing
or only gasping
and check pulse
(simultaneously).
Is pulse definitely felt
within 10 seconds?

Normal breathing, has pulse → Activate emergency response system (if not already done). Return to victim and monitor until emergency responders arrive.

No normal breathing, has pulse → Provide rescue breathing:
1 breath every 3 - 5 seconds, or about 12 - 20 breaths/min
- Add compressions if pulse remains ≤60/min with signs of poor perfusion.
- Activate emergency response system (if not already done) after 2 minutes.
- Continue rescue breathing; check pulse about every 2 minutes. If no pulse, begin CPR (go to **CPR** box).

No breathing or only gasping, no pulse

Witnessed sudden collapse? — **Yes** → Activate emergency response system (if not already done), and retrieve AED/defibrillator

No

CPR
1 rescuer: Begin cycles of 30 compressions and 2 breaths.
(Use 15:2 ratio if second rescuer arrives.) Use AED as soon as it is available

After about 2 minutes, if still alone, activate emergency response system and retrieve AED (if not already done).

Check rhythm. Shockable rhythm?

Yes, shockable → Give 1 shock. Resume CPR immediately for about 2 minutes (until prompted by AED to allow rhythm check). Continue until ALS providers take over or victim starts to move.

No, nonshockable → Resume CPR immediately for about 2 minutes (until prompted by AED to allow rhythm check). Continue until ALS providers take over or victim starts to move.

AHA (2015) Update

5. BLS Healthcare Provider Pediatric Cardiac Arrest Algorithm (2 or More Rescuers)

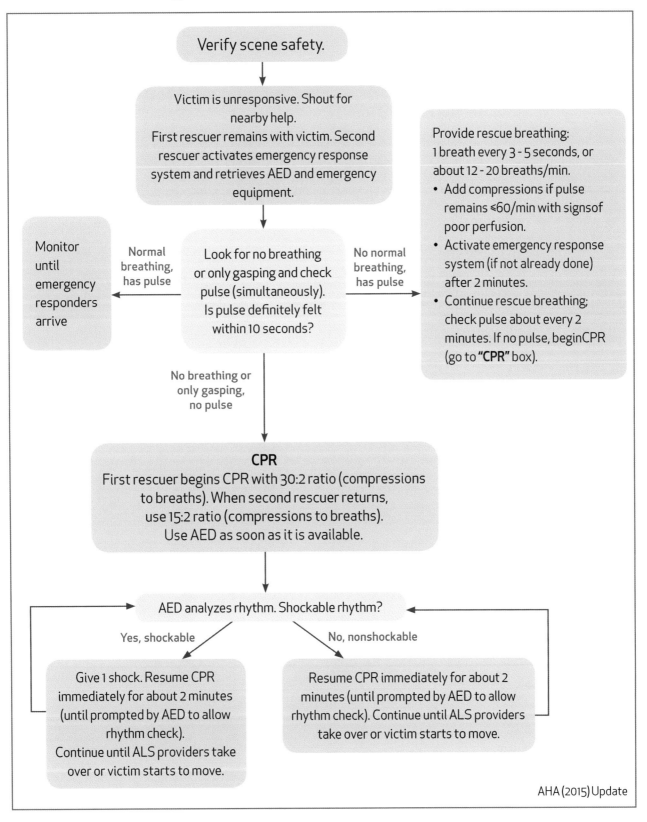

Verify scene safety.

Victim is unresponsive. Shout for nearby help.
First rescuer remains with victim. Second rescuer activates emergency response system and retrieves AED and emergency equipment.

Look for no breathing or only gasping and check pulse (simultaneously). Is pulse definitely felt within 10 seconds?

Normal breathing, has pulse → Monitor until emergency responders arrive

No normal breathing, has pulse →

Provide rescue breathing:
1 breath every 3 - 5 seconds, or about 12 - 20 breaths/min.
- Add compressions if pulse remains ≤60/min with signs of poor perfusion.
- Activate emergency response system (if not already done) after 2 minutes.
- Continue rescue breathing; check pulse about every 2 minutes. If no pulse, begin CPR (go to **"CPR"** box).

No breathing or only gasping, no pulse

CPR
First rescuer begins CPR with 30:2 ratio (compressions to breaths). When second rescuer returns, use 15:2 ratio (compressions to breaths).
Use AED as soon as it is available.

AED analyzes rhythm. Shockable rhythm?

Yes, shockable

No, nonshockable

Give 1 shock. Resume CPR immediately for about 2 minutes (until prompted by AED to allow rhythm check).
Continue until ALS providers take over or victim starts to move.

Resume CPR immediately for about 2 minutes (until prompted by AED to allow rhythm check). Continue until ALS providers take over or victim starts to move.

AHA (2015) Update

6. AHA (2015) CPR Guidelines (General BLS - Adult)

CPR should be started if the person is not responding to rescuers and does not appear to be breathing.

1. CPR begins with compressions delivered hard and fast in the middle of the person's chest. The rescuer should place the heel of one hand on the center of the person's chest and the other hand right on top of the first with fingers intertwined

2. Each compression should be at least 2" deep and delivered at a rate of at least 100/minute. After giving 30 compressions a rescuer who is able to breathe for the person should do so. If a rescuer is unable to breathe for the person they should provide continuous high quality compressions until professional rescuers arrive

3. Breaths for the person start by adjusting their airway. Tilt the person's head by the forehead back and lifting the chin to open the airway. Pinch shut the patient's nose using the forefinger and thumb

4. Each breath given to the person should be a normal breath for the rescuer and delivered over 1 second while looking for the person's chest to rise

5. A total of two breaths should be given to the person and then the rescuer should immediately start chest compressions again

6. The cycle of 30 compressions and 2 breaths should be continued until the rescuer is physically unable to do so or professional rescuers arrive

7. As soon as an AED becomes available it should be turned on and its instructions followed to connect it to the person. An AED will only work on someone who will benefit from it and will not harm someone who will not benefit from it.

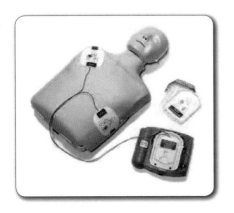

7. How to Operate an Automated External Defibrillator

1. Turn on the defibrillator. A computer - generated voice will talk through the steps

2. Place a set of adhesive electrode pads on the patient's bare chest and attach the pads' connector into the defibrillator

3. Use appropriate electrode pads i.e. Adult or Paediatric accordingly

4. The defibrillator will begin to automatically analyse the person's heart rhythm to determine if a shock is required

5. It is important that no contact be made with the person while the defibrillator is analysing the heart rhythm. If the person is touched or disturbed, the test may not be accurate

6. If the defibrillator determines that a shock is necessary, it will automatically charge itself and tell the rescuer when to press the button that will deliver the shock

7. Once the shock is delivered, or if no shock is deemed necessary, the rescuer will be prompted to check to see if the person has had a return of normal breathing or circulation.

8. If not the rescuer(s) will be reminded to start CPR

8. Anaphylaxis Guidelines

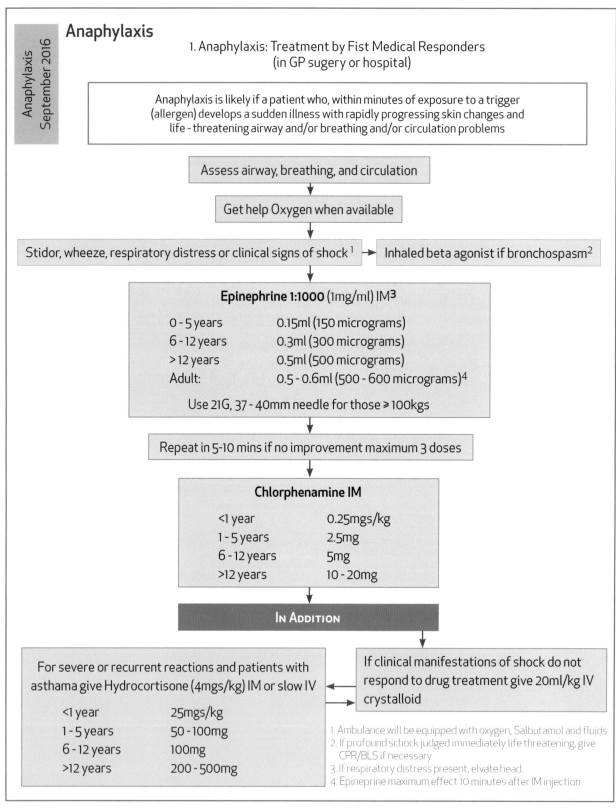

Anaphylaxis

Anaphylaxis
September 2016

1. Anaphylaxis: Treatment by Fist Medical Responders
(in GP sugery or hospital)

Anaphylaxis is likely if a patient who, within minutes of exposure to a trigger (allergen) develops a sudden illness with rapidly progressing skin changes and life - threatening airway and/or breathing and/or circulation problems

Assess airway, breathing, and circulation

Get help Oxygen when available

Stidor, wheeze, respiratory distress or clinical signs of shock [1] → Inhaled beta agonist if bronchospasm [2]

Epinephrine 1:1000 (1mg/ml) IM [3]

0 - 5 years	0.15ml (150 micrograms)
6 - 12 years	0.3ml (300 micrograms)
>12 years	0.5ml (500 micrograms)
Adult:	0.5 - 0.6ml (500 - 600 micrograms) [4]

Use 21G, 37 - 40mm needle for those ≥ 100kgs

Repeat in 5-10 mins if no improvement maximum 3 doses

Chlorphenamine IM

<1 year	0.25mgs/kg
1 - 5 years	2.5mg
6 - 12 years	5mg
>12 years	10 - 20mg

IN ADDITION

For severe or recurrent reactions and patients with asthama give Hydrocortisone (4mgs/kg) IM or slow IV

<1 year	25mgs/kg
1 - 5 years	50 - 100mg
6 - 12 years	100mg
>12 years	200 - 500mg

If clinical manifestations of shock do not respond to drug treatment give 20ml/kg IV crystalloid

1. Ambulance will be equipped with oxygen, Salbutamol and fluids
2. If profound schock judged immediately life threatening, give CPR/BLS if necessary
3. If respiratory distress present, elvate head.
4. Epineprine maximum effect 10 minutes after IM injection

Source: Health Service Executive (2016). Directions for Nurses and Midwives for the Management of a Patient who Develops Anaphylaxis and Medicine Protocol for the Administration of Epinephrine (Adrenaline) Injection BP 1: 1,000 by IM Injection by Registered Nurses and Midwives. HSE: Dublin

2. Anaphylaxis: Treatment in the Community

Anaphylaxis is likely if a patient who, within minutes of exposure to a trigger (allegen), develops a sudden illness with rapidly progressing skin changes and life - theatening airway and/or breathing and/or circulation problems

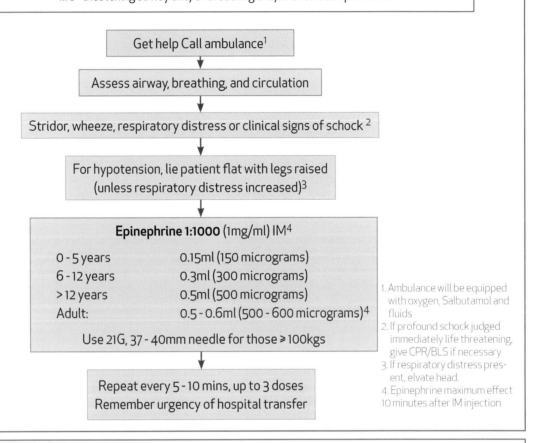

Get help Call ambulance[1]

Assess airway, breathing, and circulation

Stridor, wheeze, respiratory distress or clinical signs of schock [2]

For hypotension, lie patient flat with legs raised (unless respiratory distress increased)[3]

Epinephrine 1:1000 (1mg/ml) IM[4]

0 - 5 years	0.15ml (150 micrograms)
6 - 12 years	0.3ml (300 micrograms)
>12 years	0.5ml (500 micrograms)
Adult:	0.5 - 0.6ml (500 - 600 micrograms)[4]

Use 21G, 37 - 40mm needle for those ≥ 100kgs

Repeat every 5 - 10 mins, up to 3 doses
Remember urgency of hospital transfer

1. Ambulance will be equipped with oxygen, Salbutamol and fluids
2. If profound schock judged immediately life threatening, give CPR/BLS if necessary
3. If respiratory distress present, elvate head.
4. Epinephrine maximum effect 10 minutes after IM injection

3. Suggested Anaphylaxis Kit

The availability of protocols, equipment and drugs necessary forthe management of anaphylaxis shoulde be checked before each vaccination session

- Copy of "Anaphylaxis : Treatment in the Community" from immunisation Guidelines for Ireland
- 3x1 ml ampoules of epinephrine (1:1000, 1mg/ml)
- 6 x Epinephrine auto - injectors, 300 mcg and/or 3x500mcg* (depending on age of vacinees)

- 3x1 ml syringes
- Neeles 3x16mm, 3x25mm, 3x37 - 40mm
- 1 pocket mask
- sphygmomanometer (optional)
- Stethoscope (optional)
- Pen and paper to record time of administration of epinephrine

The kits should be kept closed to ensure the drugs are not exposed to light and stored at room temperature. The kits require regular checking to replace drugs before their expiry date.

*: Ensure that 500mcg auto - injectors have 25mm needles

Source: Health Service Executive (2016). Directions for Nurses and Midwives for the Management of a Patient who Develops Anaphylaxis and Medicine Protocol for the Administration of Epinephrine (Adrenaline) Injection BP 1: 1,000 by IM Injection by Registered Nurses and Midwives. HSE: Dublin.

9. Management of acute Adult Asthma in General Practice Protocol

Admit to hospital if any:

- Life threatening feature
- Features of acute severe asthma present after initial assessment
- Previous near fatal asthma

Lower threshold for admission if afternoon or evening attack, recent nocturnal symptoms or hospital admission, previous severe attacks, patient unable to assess own condition, or concern over social circumstances

Assess and record:

- Peak expiratory flow
- Symptoms and response to self treatment
- Heart, respiratory rates and BP
- Oxygen Saturation (by pulse oximetry, if available)

Caution

Patients with severe or life threatening attacks may not be distressed and may not have all the abnormalities listed below. The presence of any should alert the doctor. Regard each emergency asthma consultation as for acute life threatening/ severe asthma until it is shown otherwise

Life threatening Asthma	Acute severe Asthma	Moderate Asthma	Mild Asthma
Initial assessment			
Pef < 33% Best or predicted	Pef 33–50% best or predicted	Pef 50–75% best or predicted	Pef >75% best or predicted
further assessment			
- SpO2 <92% - Silent chest, cyanosis, poor respiratory effort - Bradycardia, arrhythmia, hypotension - Exhaustion, confusion, coma	- PEF <50% (severe) - Respiration >25 breaths/min - Pulse >110 beats/min - Cannot complete sentence in one breath	- Talks in phrases - RR <25 breaths/min - PR<110 beats/min - Prefer to sit - Loud wheeze	- Speech normal - RR <20 breaths/min - PR <100 beats/min - Can lie down - Mild - mod wheeze
Management			
Arrange immediate ED referral	Consider admission	Treat at home or in the surgery Assess response to treatment	

Life threatening Asthma	Acute severe Asthma	Moderate Asthma	Mild Asthma
Treatment			
- Oxygen 40–60% or higher if available - prednisolone 40–50mg or IV hydrocortisone 100mg immediately - High dose ß$_2$ bronchodilator and ipratropium: - Ideally via oxygen driven nebuliser (salbutamol 5mg or terbutaline 10mg) and ipratropium 0.5mg - OR via spacer (up to 12 puffs [given one at a time and inhaled separately]. Assess response in 10–20 mins and repeat as necessary (3 doses in total)	Oxygen 40–60% if available Maximise the dose of ß$_2$ bronchodilator: - via nebuliser (Ideally oxygen driven) salbutamol 5mg or terbutaline 10mg - OR via spacer up to 12 puffs [given one at a time and inhaled separately] Assess reponse in 10–20 mins and repeat as necessary (3 doses in total). If PEF >50-75% predicted/best - prednisolone 40–50mg or IVhydrocortisone 100mg If no response in acute severe asthma: **ADMIT** If good response to first nebulised treatment (symptoms improved, respiration and pulse rate settling and PEF >50%) continue step up usual treatment and continue prednisolone	Maximise the dose of ß$_2$ bronchodilator: - via spacer (up to 12 puffs [given one at a time and inhaled separately] Assess response in 10–20 mins and repeat as necessary (3 doses in total) - or via oxygen driven nebuliser (salbutamol 5mg or terbutaline 10mg) PEF >50–75% predicted/best: - prednisolone 40–50mg or IV hydrocortisone 100mg If good response to first nebulised treatment (symptoms improved, respiration and pulse rate settling and PEF >75%) continue step up usual treatment and continue prednisolone	- Give up to 12 puffs of regular MDI bronchodilator via spacer - Prescribe inhaled steroid - Follow - up treatment as per GINA guidelines

If admitting the patient to hospital

- Stay with patient until ambulance arrives
- Send written assessment and referral details to hospital
- Give high dose ß$_2$ bronchodilator via oxygen driven nebuliser in ambulance

Post Discharge

- GP review within 2 working days
- Address potential preventable contributors to admission
- Ensure referral to Asthma/ Respiratory Service for follow up if patient uncontrolled at step 3 (ref:GINA)
- In all patients who received nebulised ß$_2$ agonists consider an extended observation period prior to discharge home

- If PEF<50% predicted/best on presentation, prescribe prednisolone 40mg/day for 5 days. Ensure all patients have a treatment supply
- In all patients ensure prescription of inhaled steroid and ß$_2$ agonist as a minimum
- Written Asthma Management Plan with monitoring of symptoms and PEF
- Check Inhaler and peak flow meter technique
- Modify treatment according to guidelines
- Follow up within 48 hours for moderate and within 2 weeks for mild

10. Management of Acute Asthma in Children in General Practice

1. Aged 2–5 years

Life threatening asthma	Severe exacerbation	Mild/Moderate exacerbation
Assess asthma severity		
- SpO2 <92% - Silent chest - Poor respiratory effort - Agitation - Altered conciousness - Cyanosis	- SpO2 <92% - Too breathless to talk - Heart rate >130/min - Respiratory rate >50/min - Use of accessory neck muscles	- SpO2 >+92% - Able to talk - Heart rate <130/min - Respiratory rate <50/min
Treatment		

- Oxygen via facemask if available
Nebulise:
  - Salbutamol 2.5mg
  - Or terbutaline 5mg
    +
  - Ipratropium 0.25mg
  - Soluble prednisolone 20mg or IV hydrocortisone 50mg
	- Oxygen via facemask if available
	- Up to 6puffs of ß$_2$ agonist via spacer (given one at a time and inhaled separately). Review and repeat if necessary (3 doses in total) or nebulised salbutamol 2.5mg or terbutaline 5mg.
	- Soluble prednisolone 20mg
	
	Assess response to treatment 10 - 20 minutes after ß$_2$ agonist
		- ß$_2$ agonist up to 6 puffs via spacer + - facemask. Review and repeat if necessary (3 doses in total).
		- Consider soluble prednisolone 20mg
		
		Assess response to treatment 10 - 20 minutes after ß$_2$ agonist

Management		
Repeat ß$_2$ agonist via oxygen - driven nebuliser whilst arranging immediate admission to hospital	If poor response repeat ß$_2$ agonist and arrange admission	If poor response repeat ß$_2$ agonist and Arrange admission

Poor response		Good response	
- Reassess at 10 - 20 min intervals - Administer ß$_2$ agonist according to response to treatment while awaiting transfer to hospital - Stay with patient until ambulance arrives - Send written assessment and referral details - Repeat ß$_2$ agonist via oxygen - driven nebuliser in ambulance		- Continue ß$_2$ agonist via spacer or nebuliser, as needed but not exceeding 4 - hourly - If symptoms are not controlled repeat ß$_2$ agonist and refer to hospital - Continue prednisolone for up to 3 days - Arrange follow - up after 48 hours	

> ## Lower threshold for admission if
> - Attack in late afternoon or at night
> - Recent hospital admission or previous severe attack
> - Concern over social circumstances or ability to cope at home
>
> **NB:** if a patient has signs and symptoms across categories, always treat according to their most severe features

2. Aged 6–15 years

Life threatening asthma	Severe exacerbation	Mild/Moderate exacerbation
Assess asthma severity		
- SpO2 <92% - PEF <33% best or predicted - Silent chest - Poor respiratory effort - Agitation - Altered conciousness - Cyanosis	- SpO2 <92% - PEF < 50% best or predicted - Too breathless to talk - Heart rate >120/min - Respiratory rate >30/min - Use of accessory neck muscles	- SpO2 ≥ 92% - PEF ≥50% best or predicted - Able to talk - Heart rate ≤120/min - Respiratory rate <30/min
Treatment		

- Oxygen via facemask if available
  Nebulise:
    - Salbutamol 5mg
    - Orterbutaline 10mg
    +
    - Ipratropium 0.25mg
    - Soluble prednisolone
    30–40mg or IV hydrocortisone
    100mg
	- Oxygen via facemask if available
	- Up to 12 puffs of β_2 agonist via spacer (given one at a time and inhaled separately). Review and repeat if necessary after 20mins (3 doses in total). or nebulised salbutamol 2.5–5mg or terbutaline 5–10mg.
	- Soluble prednisolone 30–40mg
	
	Assess response to treatment 10 - 20 minutes after β_2 agonist
		- β_2 agonist up to 12 puffs via spacer + facemask. Review and repeat if necessary after 20mins (3 doses in total).
		- Consider soluble prednisolone 30–40mg
		
		Assess response to treatment 10 - 20 minutes after β_2 agonist

Management		
Repeat β_2 agonist via oxygen - driven nebuliser while arranging immediate hospital admission	If poor response repeat β_2 agonist and arrange admission	If poor response repeat β_2 agonist and Arrange admission
Poor response		**Good response**
- Reassess at 10–20 min intervals - Administer β_2 agonist according to response to treatment while awaiting transfer to hospital - Stay with patient until ambulance arrives - Send written assessment and referral details - Repeat β_2 agonist via oxygen - driven nebuliser in ambulance		- Continue β_2 agonist via spacer or nebuliser, as needed but not exceeding 4 - hourly - If symptoms are not controlled repeat β_2 agonist and refer to hospital - Continue prednisolone for up to 3 days - Arrange follow - up after 48 hours

Lower threshold for admission if
- Attack in late afternoon or at night
- Recent hospital admission or previous severe attack
- Concern over social circumstances or ability to cope at home

NB: if a patient has signs and symptoms across categories, always treat according to their most severe features

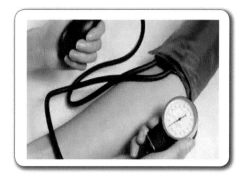

11. Blood Pressure Measurement (Manual)

Equipment

- Sphygmomanometer
- Stethoscope
- Range of cuff sizes
- Alcohol hand - rub
- Detergent/antiseptic wipes

Procedure

1. Explain the procedure and gain informed consent

2. Decontaminate hands using correct hand hygiene techniques

3. Ask and observe the patient for any of the following
   - Lymphoedema
   - Arteriovenous fistula
   - Trauma or surgery to arm or axilla
   - Brachial artery surgery
   - Implant

4. If there is a contraindication, use the other arm or if bilateral, the lower extremity

5. The patient should be seated comfortably for at least five minutes prior to measuring BP

6. Choose the correct size cuff for the arm

7. Check the patients arm is free from clothing, supported and placed at heart level

8. Wrap the cuff of the sphygmomanometer around the bare upper arm with the centre over the brachial artery and superior to the elbow. The lower edge of the cuff should be 2 - 3 cm above the brachial artery pulsation

9. Ask the patient not to talk during the procedure

10. Inflate the cuff to 20 - 30 mmHg above the predicted systolic blood pressure

11. Release the air in the cuff slowly until the first tapping sounds are heard (first Korotkoff sound). This is the systolic blood pressure

12. Continue to deflate the cuff slowly, listening to the Korotkoff sounds; the point at which the sound completely disappears is the best representation of the diastolic blood pressure (fifth Korotkoff sound)

13. Once sound can no longer be heard, rapidly deflate the cuff

14. If necessary to re - check the BP, wait 1 - 2 minutes before proceeding

15. Inform patient that the procedure is now finished

16. Decontaminate hands using correct hand hygiene techniques

17. Clean bell and diaphragm of stethoscope

18. Document the recording (s) in the patients notes

19. Compare with previous results, take action as appropriate.

12. Pulse Measurement Guidelines

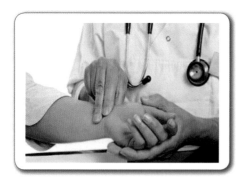

Equipment

- Watch with a second hand or
- Electronic pulse measurement device i.e.
- pulse oximeter or blood pressure monitor
- Stethescope if counting the apical beat
- Alcohol hand - rub
- Patient's notes

Procedure

1. Explain the procedure to the patient and gain informed consent
2. Decontaminate hands using correct hand hygiene techniques
3. Where possible measure the pulse under the same conditions each time
4. Ensure the patient is comfortable and relaxed. Ideally the patient should refrain from physical activity for 20 minutes before the pulse is measured
5. The pulse rate may be recorded via an electronic devise such as a pulse oximeter applied to the finger or via an electronic blood pressure monitoring device
6. For manual pulse measurement: Place the first and second or in addition the third finger along the appropriate artery (usually the radial artery) and apply light pressure until the pulse is felt
7. Press gently against the peripheral artery being used to record the pulse
8. If the apical heart rate requires recording, place a stethoscope on the left mid - clavicle, 4th - 5th intercostal space or left midclavicular line (typically under the breast) and listen to the heartbeat
9. The pulse should be counted for 60 seconds
10. Record the pulse rate on the patients notes, including any comments regarding the rhythm, volume and skin condition
11. Discuss the result and any further action (if required) with the patient
12. Wash and dry hands and decontaminate the stethoscope with an alcohol wipe

13. Temperature Measurement (Tympanic)

Equipment

- Tympanic membrane thermometer
- Disposable probe covers
- Alcohol hand - rub

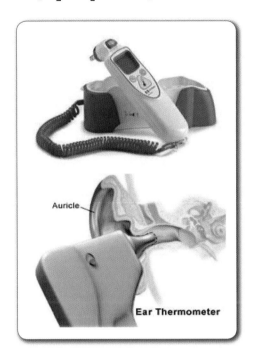

Auricle

Ear Thermometer

Procedure

1. Explain the procedure and gain informed consent

2. If the patient is wearing a hearing aid, remove the device from the ear and wait 10 minutes before taking a reading

3. Decontaminate hands using correct hand hygiene techniques

4. Inspect the outer ear canal for any drainage, discharge or foreign body

5. Remove the thermometer from the base unit and ensure the probe lens is calibrated clean and intact

6. Depending on the model of thermometer, verify the mode setting on the LCD display to show the route of measurement (example ear) if applicable

7. Place disposable probe cover on the probe tip

8. Obtain a reading from both ears and use the greater of the readings

9. A new probe cover must be used for each reading to ensure the highest degree of accuracy and to prevent cross contamination between ears

10. Ensure the patient has not been lying on their ear 20 minutes prior to recording the temperature. If the patient has been lying on one ear, take the temperature in the exposed ear.

11. Align the probe with the ear canal and gently advance into the ear canal, until the probe lightly seals the opening, ensuring a snug fit

12. Press and release the scan button

13. Remove probe tip from the ear when the thermometer displays the temperature reading, usually indicated by a bleep

14. Document the reading on the patient's records.

15. Take action as appropriate if temperature is abnormal

16. Press the release/ eject button to remove cover from probe and dispose of in clinical waste

17. Clean the thermometer as per manufacturers guidelines

18. Decontaminate hands using correct hand hygiene techniques

14. Pulse Oximetry Guidelines

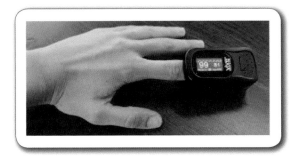

Pulse Oximetry is a non - invasive method that enables rapid measurement of the oxygen saturation of hemoglobin in arterial blood. Pulse Oximetry can rapidly detect changes in oxygen saturation, thus providing an early warning of hypoxaemia (insufficient oxygen content in the blood)

Contraindications

Pulse oximetry does not give an indication of haemoglobin so if the patient is profoundly anaemic then their oxygen saturation may be normal but they may still be hypoxic.

Equipment

- Pulse Oximeter
- Medicated cleaning wipes
- Patient Documentation/Health records

Procedure

1. Explain the procedure and gain informed consent

2. Whilst talking to the patient assess their respiratory condition including their ability to talk in full sentences, the colour of their skin, whether they appear to be in distress or not, and whether they are alert and orientated

3. Ensure the probe is clean and is in good working order

4. Decontaminate hands using correct hand hygiene techniques

5. Select a suitable area for the probe (usually fingertip), ensure the correct size of probe is utilized e.g. adults or children

6. Switch the pulse oximeter machine on, make sure that the probe sensor is detecting the pulse. This will usually be indicated by a beep in time with each detected pulse or a graphical indication of the pulse on a display panel

7. Once oxygen saturation monitoring is complete, remove the probe and ensure patient is comfortable

8. Record oxygen saturation in the patient's record and inform patient. Record the flow/concentration of any current oxygen therapy in litres per minute if applicable.

9. Record if the measurement was taken with the patient at rest or walking

10. If the reading is outside the patient's parameters: Check the oximeter is working correctly. Reassure the patient and report any abnormalities

11. Explain results to patient and any necessary action needed to change current treatment plan if required. Document all actions in patient's record

12. Decontaminate hands and clean the pulse oximeter according to manufacturer's recommendations

15. Measuring Peak Flow Using a Manual Peak Flow Meter

Peak expiratory flow (PEF) is the highest flow achieved on forced expiration from a position of maximum lung inflation expressed in litres per minute (L/min).

Equipment

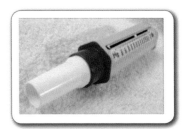

- Peak Flow Meter Disposable Mouthpiece
- Peak flow chart and pen to record results
- Pulse Oximetry (if required)
- Oxygen Mask and Oxygen source (If required)
- Equipment to give a nebuliser (if required)
- Emergency resuscitation equipment (available if required

Procedure

1. Ask the patient what their best peak flow measurements have been and what their current peak flow readings are
2. Decontaminate hands using correct hand hygiene techniques
3. Assemble equipment: ask the patient to use their own meter, if it is in good working order and less than 1 year old
4. If using a multiple patient device, ensure that it has been cleaned and use a new single use disposable mouthpiece
5. Position the patient sitting upright or preferably standing
6. Ensure indicator is at bottom of scale, i.e. zero (0)
7. Ask the patient to hold the peak flow meter horizontally, ensuring their fingers do not impede the gauge
8. Ask the patient to take a deep breath in, and then to place their lips tightly around the mouthpiece
9. Ask the patient to blow out as quickly and hard as possible, to push the pointer up the scale
10. Note the reading and return the pointer on the gauge to zero
11. Allow the patient a moment to rest and then repeat the procedure twice, recording the readings each time

12. Ideally there should be less than 20L/min difference between the three readings. If there is more than 40 L/min difference in the recordings, two additional blows can be performed

13. Document the highest of the three acceptable readings

14. Document the readings on the patients chart, comparing measured values against predicted values or patient trends and report any abnormality

15. Dispose of the mouthpiece in the clinical waste and clean the meter in line with policies and manufacturers recommendations

16. Decontaminate hands using correct hand hygiene techniques

Infection control

Meters must be restricted to single patient use only to prevent any risks of cross infection. In areas where meters are shared, disposable mouthpieces must be used and particular attention paid to cleaning the meter after use.

The plastic meters should be washed in hot water with detergent, rinsed or wiped with universal sanitizing wipes and dried thoroughly at least once a week

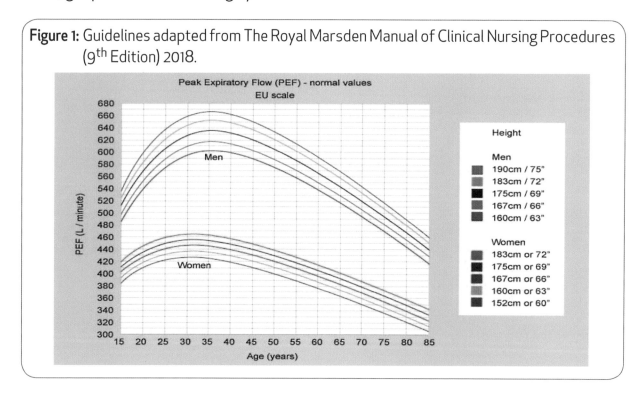

Figure 1: Guidelines adapted from The Royal Marsden Manual of Clinical Nursing Procedures (9th Edition) 2018.

16. Urinalysis Reagent Strip Guidelines

Equipment

- Non - sterile disposable gloves
- Apron
- Urine reagent sticks Urine specimen jar

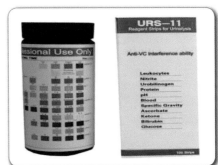

Procedure

1. Explain the procedure to the patient and gain informed consent

2. Decontaminate hands using correct hand hygiene techniques, and apply gloves and apron

3. Provide a urine specimen jar and ask the patient to attend the bathroom to provide a sample of midstream urine. Explain that they should commence micturition into the toilet and when a few millimetres of urine has been passed into the toilet, catch a flow of urine into the specimen jar and when filled to pass any remaining urine into the toilet

4. Check reagent strips are in date and have been stored in accordance with manufacturer's instructions

5. Dip the reagent strip into the urine. The strip should be completely immersed in the urine and then removed immediately. Run the edge of the strip along the container

6. Hold the stick at an angle

7. Wait the required time (usually 60 seconds) before reading the strip against the colour chart

8. Dispose of urine sample appropriately in sluice or toilet. Dispose of urinalysis stick and gloves in the clinical waste. Ensure the cap of the reagent strips is replaced immediately and closed tightly

9. Decontaminate hands using correct hand hygiene techniques

10. Document the urinalysis reading, discuss result with the patient and report/ follow up on any abnormal reading

---

Note: If taking the sample from a urinary catheter, the sample should be collected using aseptic techniques via the catheter side port

17. Blood Glucose Meter Monitoring Guidelines

Equipment

- Blood glucose meter
- Glucose test strips
- Single use sampling device
- Paper towel & tissue
- Non - sterile gloves
- Sharps bin

Procedure

1. Explain the procedure to the patient and gain informed consent

2. Ensure machine is calibrated using corresponding code chip to match strip lot number

3. Ensure meter has quality control (QC) performed. This should be done as a minimum weekly or daily if using for more than one patient such as in a clinic, or before each single use, and when new box of strips started. If opening a new QC solution, record the date on the pot(s) and expiry date. Record the QC result in the meter Quality control record book

4. Ask the patient to wash their hands with soap and warm water, and dry thoroughly

5. Decontaminate hands according to correct hand hygiene techniques and put on gloves

6. Protect work surface with paper towel

7. Where the meter requires coding, ensure that the code number on the meter display matches that on the test strip

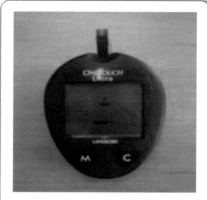
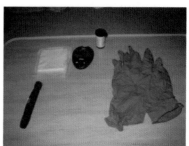
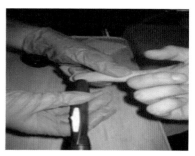
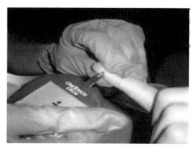

8. Check expiry dates of test strips

9. Remove strip from container and insert into the meter

10. Use single use lancet sampling device and discard sampling device in sharps bin after use

11. Prick side of finger (avoid finger pad, thumb and index finger where possible) wait 10 - 20 seconds and, if drop of blood has not appeared, gently 'milk' finger if necessary by massaging finger from base towards fingertip to help with blood circulation to fingertip ensuring hand is below heart level

12. Take the strip in the meter to the blood and ensuring meter and strip are above the drop of blood touch the strip tip into the blood

13. Wait until the meter displays the blood glucose reading

14. Wipe away any blood, with tissue, from the patient's finger

15. Remove and safely dispose of test strip from meter in clinical waste

16. Remove gloves and clean hands using correct hand hygiene techniques

17. Document result in patient's notes

18. If glucose result is outside target range take appropriate action

19. The blood glucose monitoring device must be cleaned prior to use on another patient

18. ECG Lead Placement Guidelines

There are 10 wires on an ECG machine connected to specific parts of the body. A lead is a view of electrical activity of the heart from a specific angle across the body. Even though there are only 10 leads, the ECG provides 12 views from different angles. Hence the name 12 lead ECG.

These wires break down into 2 groups:

1.　6 chest leads
2.　4 limb or peripheral leads (one of these is "neutral")

The 6 chest leads are positioned as below

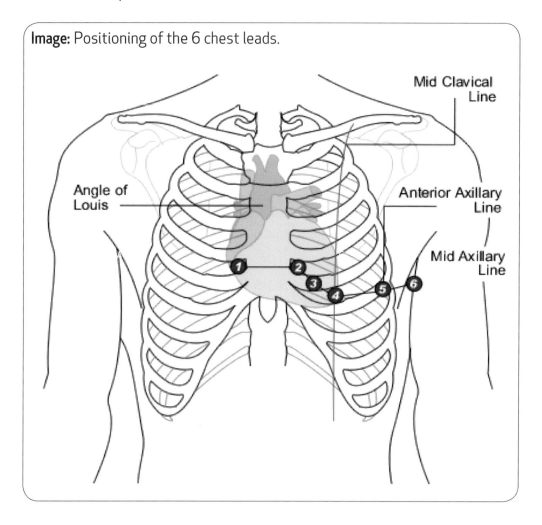

Image: Positioning of the 6 chest leads.

Limb Leads

Limb leads are made up of 4 leads placed on the extremities: left and right wrist; left and right ankle.

The lead connected to the right ankle is a neutral lead. It is there to complete an electrical circuit and plays no role in the ECG itself.

Electrode Placement

Electrode	Placement
V1	4th Intercostal space at the right sternal edge
V2	4th Intercostal space at the left sternal edge
V3	Midway between V2 and V4
V4	5th Intercostal space at the midclavicular line
V5	Left anterior axillary line at the same horizontal level as V4
V6	Left mid - axillary line at the same horizontal level as V4 and V5
RL (Black)	Right lower leg, proximal to the ankle
RA (Red)	Right forearm, proximal to the wrist
LL (Green)	Left lower leg, proximal to the ankle
LA (Yellow)	Left forearm, proximal to the wrist
Source: Society for Cardiological Science and Technology (2014). Clinical Guidelines by Consensus. Recording a Standard 12 Lead Electrocardiogram. SCST: UK	

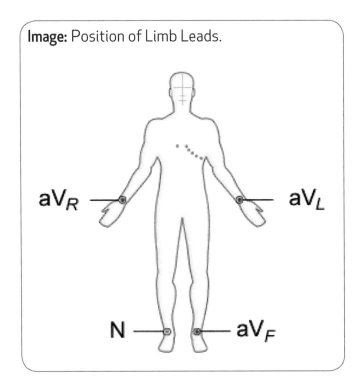

Image: Position of Limb Leads.

19. Recording an Electrocardiogram (ECG)

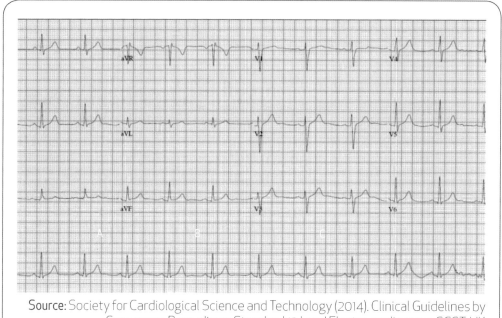

Source: Society for Cardiological Science and Technology (2014). Clinical Guidelines by Consensus. Recording a Standard 12 Lead Electrocardiogram. SCST: UK

Equipment

- 12 lead ECG machine with chest and limb leads labelled respectively
- Disposable electrodes
- Alcohol hand rub

Procedure

1. Explain the procedure to the patient and gain informed consent
2. Decontaminate hands according to correct hand hygiene techniques
3. Ensure privacy and that the patient is positioned comfortably in the semi - recumbent position with chest and limbs exposed
4. Any variations to standard recording techniques must be highlighted on the ECG recording and in the patients notes (example ECG recorded whilst patient in wheelchair)
5. Ensure skin is clean and if necessary body hair may be clipped/ shaved
6. Apply the limb and chest electrodes (as explained/ shown above)
7. Attach the cables from the ECG machine to the electrodes checking that the cables are connected correctly to the relevant electrodes

8. Ensure that the cables are not pulling on the electrodes or lying over each other. Offer the patient a sheet or cover to place over their exposed chest

9. Ask patient to relax and refrain from movement

10. Encourage patient to breathe normally and not to speak while the recording is being taken

11. Switch the machine on and enter the patients details into the machine

12. Check that the machine is functioning correctly and that calibration is 10mm/mV

13. Commence the recording

14. In case of artefact or poor recording, check electrodes and connections

15. Once complete, detach the ECG printout and ensure the recording is labelled with the patients' name, patient number, date and time. Also include any diagnostic information (i.e. if any chest pain during the recording) and deviation to the standard electrode placement

16. If the ECG is irregular or abnormal, record a 10 second rhythm strip, usually from lead II

17. Inform the patient that the procedure is complete and help to remove the electrodes

18. Decontaminate hands using correct hand hygiene techniques

19. Show the ECG recording to the Doctor for review/ analysis

20. File the recording in the appropriate patient documentation

21. Clean the ECG machine in accordance with manufacturer's recommendations. Return to its storage place and plug into the mains electricity to keep the battery fully charged

20. Assessing Fractures Guidelines 5 P's

The "5 P's

1. Pain
2. Pulse
3. Pallor
4. Paresthesia
5. Paralysis

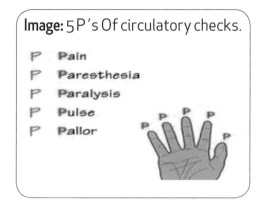

Image: 5 P's Of circulatory checks.

P   Pain
P   Paresthesia
P   Paralysis
P   Pulse
P   Pallor

All nursing assessment findings should be documented in the patient's chart so that comparison can be made with notes made at both earlier and later dates. In this way, the patient's progress can be followed and changes in status are easily recognized..

In addition to the five P's mentioned above, the patient's level of consciousness and temperature should be checked regularly.

Mental status changes and temperature elevation could indicate the presence of infection. Reposition the patient as necessary to relieve pressure areas.

Check all dressings, bandages, casts, splints, and traction equipment to ensure that nothing is causing constriction or pressure.

Frequent and thorough checking and observation on the part of the nursing staff will promote healing and prevent complications.

Life Threatening Complications

Pulmonary Embolism

Is the occlusion of the pulmonary arteries by a thrombus originating in the venous system. Patients with lower extremity fractures are most susceptible to pulmonary embolism

1. Pain
Determine where the pain is located and the level of pain. Worsening pain may indicate increased oedema, lack of adequate blood supply, or tissue damage

2. Pulse
Check the peripheral pulses, especially those distal to the fracture site. Compare all pulses with those on the unaffected side. Pulses should be strong and equal

3. Pallor
Observe the colour and temperature of the skin, especially around the fracture site. Perform the capillary refill (blanching) test.

4. Paresthesia
Examine the injured area for increase or decrease in sensation. Can the patient detect tactile stimulation such as a blunt touch or a sharp pinprick? Does the patient complain of numbness or tingling?

5. Paralysis
Check the patient's mobility. Can the patient wiggle their toes and fingers? Can the patient move their extremities?

21. Neurological Observations and Assessment

Equipment

- Pen torch
- Thermometer
- Sphygmomanometer
- Tongue Depressor
- Patella Hammer
- Neuro tips
- Alcohol hand - rub
- Low linting swabs
- Test tubes x 2
- Snellen chart
- Ophthalmoscope

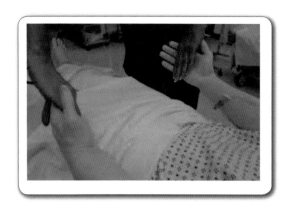

Procedure

1. Explain the procedure to the patient (whether alert or not) and attempt to gain informed consent

2. Decontaminate hands according to correct hand hygiene techniques

3. Observe the patient without speech or touch

4. Talk to the patient. Note whether they are alert and giving their full attention or restless or lethargic and drowsy. Ask the patient their name, where they are, what day, month and year it is. Also ask details about their family

5. To evaluate motor responses ask the patient to squeeze and release your fingers (both sides should be assessed) and then to stick out their tongue and raise their eyebrows

6. If the patient does not respond apply painful stimuli

7. Record the findings precisely, recording the best responses. Record exactly which stimulus was used, where it was applied, how much pressure was needed to elicit the response, and how the patient responded

8. Extend both hands and ask the patient to squeeze your fingers as hard as possible. Compare grip and strength

9. Reduce any external bright light by darkening the room, or shield the patients eyes with your hands

10. Ask the patient to open their eyes. If they cannot do so, hold the eyelids open and note the size, shape and equality of both pupils simultaneously

11. Hold each eyelid open in turn. Shine a bright light into each eye, moving from the outer corner of each eye towards the pupil. This should cause the pupil to constrict immediately and an immediate and brisk dilation of the pupil once the light is withdrawn

12. Record pupillary size (in mm) and reactions on observation chart. Brisk reaction is documented as '+' and no reaction as '-', sluggish response of one pupil compared to the other is recorded as S

13. Record unusual eye movements such as nystagmus or deviation to the side

14. Note the rate, character and pattern of the patients respirations

15. Take and record the patients temperature at specified intervals

16. Take and record the patients' blood pressure and pulse at specified intervals

17. Ask the patient to close their eyes and hold their arms straight out in front, with palms upwards for 20 – 30 seconds. Observe for any sign of weakness or drift

18. To test arm strength stand in front of the patient and extend your hands. Ask the patient to push and pull against your hands. To test flexion and extension of the extremities ask the patient to lie on their back on the bed/ couch. Place the patients legs with knees flexed and foot resting. Instruct the patient to keep the foot down as you attempt to extend the leg. Then instruct the patient to straighten the leg while you offer resistance

19. Flex and extend all the patients limbs in turn. Note how well the movements are resisted

20. To assess hand and arm co-ordination, ask the patient to pat their thigh as fast as possible. The dominant hand should perform better. Note whether the movements seem slow or clumsy. Ask the patient to turn the hand over and back several times in succession. Evaluate co-ordination. Ask the patient to touch the back of the fingers with the thumb in sequence rapidly

21. To assess hand and arm co-ordination / cerebellar function, extend one of your arms towards the patient. Ask the patient to touch your index finger, then their nose several times in succession. Repeat the test with the patients eyes closed

22. To assess leg co-ordination, ask the patient to place a heel on the opposite knee and slide it down the shin to the foot. Check each leg separately

23. To assess corneal (blink) reflex, ask the patient to look up or hold the eyelid open. With your hand, approach the eye unexpectedly or touch the eyelashes

24. To test the gag reflex, ask the patient to open their mouth and hold down the tongue with a tongue depressor. Touch the back of the pharynx on each side with a low linting swab

25. To assess the deep tendon knee jerk reflex, ask the patient to lie on their back. Place your hand under the knee, raise and flex it. Tap the patellar tendon. Note whether the leg responds

26. To assess for upper motor neurone lesion, stroke the lateral aspect of the sole of the patient's foot. If the response is abnormal (Babinski's response), the big toe will dorsiflex and the remaining toes will fan out

27. To test for visual acuity, ask the patient to read something aloud. Check each eye separately. If vision is so poor that the patient is unable to read, ask the patient to count your upraised fingers or distinguish light from dark

28. To test hearing and comprehension, occlude one ear with a low linting swab. Stand a short way from the patient. Whisper numbers into the open ear. Ask for feedback. Repeat for the other ear

29. To test superficial sensations to pain, ask the patient to close their eyes. Using the point of a neuro tip (sharp instrument for applying pressure) stroke the skin. Use the blunt end occasionally. Ask the patient to tell you what is felt. See if the patient can distinguish between sharp and dull sensation

30. To test superficial sensations to temperature, ask the patient to close their eyes. Fill two test tubes with water, one warm and one cold. Touch the patients skin with each test tube and ask the patient to distinguish between them

31. To test for superficial sensations to touch, stroke a low linting swab over the patient's skin. Ask the patient what they feel

32. To test proprioception (receipt of information from muscles and tendons in the labyrinth that enables the brain to determine movements and position of the body), ask the patient to close their eyes. Hold the tip of one of the patient's fingers between your thumb and index finger. Move it up and down and ask the patient to say in which direction it is moving. Repeat with the other hand. For the legs hold the big toe

33. Document the observation recordings on the patients observation chart. Record only what you see. Do not be influenced by previous observations

34. Report any abnormalities to the Doctor

35. Decontaminate hands using correct hand hygiene techniques

36. Clean the equipment after use according to manufacturer's guidelines

22. Glasgow Coma Scale Neurological Observation Sheet

Name:
Patient number:

Glasgow coma scale neurological observation chart

				Date
				Time

G L A S G O W C O M A S C A L E	Eyes Open	Spontaneously	4	Eyes closed by swelling = C
		To Speech	3	
		To Pain	2	
		Never	1	
	Best Verbal Response	Orientated	5	Enter a T if person has a Tracheostomy
		Confused	4	
		Inappropriate words	3	
		Incomprehensible Sounds	2	
		Silent	1	
	Best Motor Response	Obeys Commands	6	Usually record the best arm response
		Localises pain	5	
		Flexion withdrawal	4	
		Decorticate flexion	3	
		Decerebrate extension	2	
		No Response	1	
		Total		

Pupil Scale (mm)
- • 1
- • 2
- ● 3
- ● 4
- ● 5
- ● 6
- ● 7
- ● 8

Blood Pressure And Pulse Rate

240
230
220
210
200
190
180
170
160
150
140
130
120
110
100
90
80
70
60
50
40
30
Respiration 20
10

40
39
38
37
36
35
34
33
32
31
30

Pupils	Right	Size		**+** reacts − no reaction C eye closed
		Reaction		
	Left	Size		
		Reaction		

L I M B M O V E M E N T	Arms	Normal Power		Record right (R) and Left (L) separately if there is a difference between two sides
		Mild Weakness		
		Severe Weakness		
		Spastic Flexion		
		Extension		
		No response		
	Legs	Normal Power		
		Mild Weakness		
		Severe Weakness		
		Extension		
		No response		

23. The Glasgow Coma Scale

Adult Glasgow Coma Scale

The Glasgow Coma Scale (GCS) is used to describe the general level of consciousness in patients with traumatic brain injury (TBI) and to define broad categories of head injury. The GCS is divided into 3 categories, eye opening (E), motor response (M), and verbal response (V). The score is determined by the sum of the score in each of the 3 categories, with a maximum score of 15 and a minimum score of 3. GCS score = E + M + V

Response	Scale	Score Point
Eye Opening Response	Eyes open spontaneously	4
	Eyes open to verbal command, speech, or shout	3
	Eyes open to pain (not applied to face)	2
	No eye opening	1
Verbal Response	Oriented	5
	Confused conversation, but able to answer questions	4
	Inappropriate responses, words discernible	3
	Incomprehensible sounds or speech	2
	No verbal response	1
Motor Response	Obeys commands for movement	6
	Purposeful movement to painful stimulus	5
	Withdraws from pain	4
	Abnormal (spastic) flexion, decorticate posture	3
	Extensor (rigid) response, decerebrate posture	2
	No mo or response	1
Minor Brain Injury = 13 - 15 points; **Moderate Brain Injury** = 9 - 12 points; **Severe Brain Injury** = 3 - 8 points		

Interpretation

The GCS is often used to help define the severity of Traumatic Brain Injury (TBI). Mild head injuries are generally defined as those associated with a GCS score of 13 - 15, and moderate head injuries are those associated with a GCS score of 9 - 12. A GCS score of 8 or less defines a severe head injury. These definitions are not rigid and should be considered as a general guide to the level of injury.

24. Neurological Observations Chart Guidelines

A standard chart should be used to record and display neurological observations, assessments and vital signs using the Glasgow Coma Scale, pupil size and reaction and movement of limbs. Neurological observations include assessment of conscious level, vital signs, pupil size and reaction, motor response and verbal response

Glasgow Coma Scale

The Glasgow Coma Scale uses objective observable characteristics and provides a scale by which to measure level of consciousness and response. The scale is used for assessment of eye opening, best verbal response and best motor response

Eye Opening

Assessing eye opening provides an indication of the person's arousal ability. Determine if the person responds to speech (use a loud voice) or to touch. If the person does not respond, apply pressure to the finger beds to determine if there is a response to painful stimuli. If the person cannot open his or her eyes due to swelling, record 'C', or if the person's eyes remain continuously open this should be recorded as a non - eye opening response

Verbal Response

This assessment determines appropriateness of the person's speech. The person's attention should be gained and a conversation attempted, allowing adequate time for the person to respond. In assessing the person's best verbal response, consider their preferred language, any diagnosed problems that may influence their ability to respond, for example deafness, previous stroke, level of confusion prior to fall and determine if there are any changes to the person's pre - fall condition. Assess the person's response and record:

- Oriented – person can respond appropriately to person/place/time
- Confused – person can talk but is not orientated
- Inappropriate words – speaks only a few words usually in response to physical or painful stimuli
- Incomprehensible sounds – unintelligible sounds such as moans
- None – no response after prolonged stimulation

Motor Response

Assess the person using simple commands to determine if the person has the awareness/ability to respond by movement. If the person does not respond to verbal commands such as "squeeze my hands" or "open your eyes, check the person's best motor response, taking into consideration their usual level of comprehension, usual ability to move their body and any existing medical diagnoses that may contribute to their ability to move for example, previous stroke, dementia. Assess the person's response and record:

- Obeys command: follows your command
- Localises pain: moves limb away from painful stimuli in a purposeful way or attempts to push painful stimulus away
- Flexion to pain: responds to painful stimuli by bending arms up but does not localise pain
- Extension to pain – responds to painful stimuli by straightening arms but does not localise pain

Assessment of Pupils

Assessment of the person's pupil size and response to light can provide an indication as to the presence and extent of head injury as a result of a fall. The neurological observation chart should provide a pupil scale on which to assess pupil size. An assessment should first be made as to whether the person's pupils are of equal size and then whether they react equally to exposure to light

Assessment of Limb Movement

Assessment of the person's limb movement can give an indication as to the presence and extent of head injury as a result of a fall. Instruct the person to move their limbs laterally or lift up against gravity or against resistance. If the person does not respond to the request, assess limb movement in response to pain. Observe the type of movement the person can perform and compare the strength of both sides of the body. In assessing the person's limb movements and strength, consider their previous condition and any medical diagnoses that may preclude normal limb movement, for example stroke, musculoskeletal disorders. Consider whether the person has sustained injuries to the limbs, such as fractures, during the fall which may preclude normal movement. Assess and then record:

- Normal power: movements are within the person's normal power strength

- Mild weakness: cannot fully lift limbs against gravity and struggles to move against resistance

- Severe weakness: can move limbs laterally but cannot move against gravity or resistance

- Spastic flexion: arms slowly bend at elbow and are stiff

- Extension: limbs straighten

References

Bickley, L. Szilagyi, P. Hoffman, R. (2017). *Bates Guide to Physical Examination and History Taking.* 12th edn. Philadelphia: Lipincott Williams & Wilkins.

Dougherty, L. & Lister, S. (2015). The Royal Marsden Hospital Manual of Clinical Nursing Procedures. 9th Ed. Wiley Blackwell Pub: Chichester.

25. Head Injury Guidelines and Advice Sheet

Emergency symptoms

Hospital Emergency Department (A&E) immediately or phone 999

- Unconsciousness, or lack of full consciousness
- Drowsiness (feeling sleepy) that goes on for longer than 1 hour when you would normally be wide awake
- Problems understanding or speaking
- Loss of balance or problems walking
- Weakness in one or more arms or legs
- Problems with your vision
- Painful/ severe headache that won't go away
- Vomiting (being sick)
- Seizures (convulsions or fits)
- Clear fluid coming from the ear or nose
- Bleeding from one or both ears

Home Care Advice

- DO NOT stay unattended or home alone for the first 24/48 hours
- Stay within easy reach of a telephone and medical help
- DO have plenty of rest and avoid stressful situations
- Ice pack (covered) can be used to reduce any swelling (Haematoma)
- DO NOT take any alcohol or drugs
- DO NOT take sleeping pills, sedatives or tranquillisers
- Paracetamol (following correct dosage) can be taken for mild headaches if not contra - indicated or allergic to same. Seek medical advice first
- DO NOT play any contact sport (for example, rugby or football) or partake in any heavy activity for at least 3 weeks without medical advice
- DO NOT return to school, college or work until completely recovered
- DO NOT drive a car, motorbike or bicycle or operate machinery until completely recovered

Adapted from: © National Institute for Health and Care Excellence, 2014. 'Head injury', NICE clinical guideline 176.

26. Respiratory Examination Guidelines

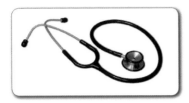

Equipment

- Stethoscope
- Examination couch

Procedure

1. Explain the procedure and gain informed consent

2. Ensure the patient is comfortable and positioned on the edge of chair or couch

3. Ensure privacy and ask the patient to remove upper garments

4. Decontaminate hands using correct hand hygiene techniques

General inspection

5. Look at the patient's skin and nails. Feel the temperature, texture and turgor of the skin

6. To assess for capillary refill press the patient's fingernail firmly for 5 seconds between your finger and thumb and then let go. Count how many seconds it takes for the colour to return to the nail

7. To assess for flapping tremor ask the patient to hold out their arms with the wrists flexed and palms facing forward for one minute

Figure 1: Ladder pattern for percussion and auscultation of the chest.

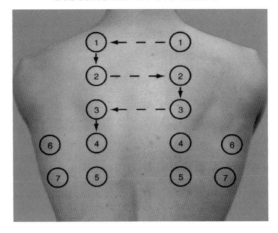

Figure 2: Location for feeling Tactile Fremitus (Anterior and Posterior views)

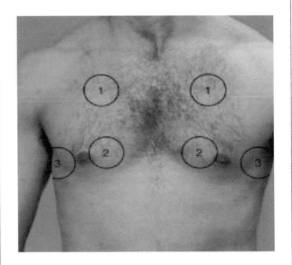

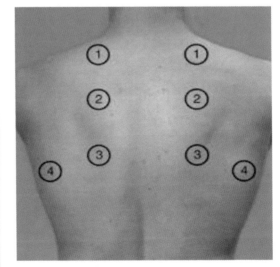

Source: Photographs courtesy of Oxford Medical Education

8. Look at the patients eyes, to assess for any abnormalities and signs of hypercholesterolaemia and anaemia

9. Look at and in the patients mouth to check for any abnormalities, sores, infection, signs of mouth breathing or URTI

10. Look at and in the patients nose to assess for nasal flare, deviated septum, polyps

11. Listen to the patients breathing to assess for any audible wheeze or stridor

12. Look at the patients neck to assess if accessory muscles are being used and if the trachea is midline

13. Palpate the trachea gently with the index finger and thumb to ensure it is midline with no deviation

14. Palpate the head and neck notes to assess for enlarged nodes

Posterior Chest

15. Inspect the patient's posterior chest to assess for scars, masses, deformities, asymmetry

16. Lightly palpate the chest to assess for signs of tenderness, pain or masses

17. To assess chest expansion place your thumbs at the level of the tenth rib either side of the spine with your fingers fanned out towards the lateral side of the chest, and ask the patient to take a deep breath in

18. To assess for tactile fremitus place the edge of your palm and little finger on the patient's chest and ask the patient to say 99

19. Percuss the chest to assess for a normal resonant lung and identifying any abnormalities

20. Auscultate the lung using the diaphragm of the stethoscope to assess for vesicular breath sounds and any adventitious sounds

Anterior Chest

1. Inspect the anterior chest to assess for any scars, masses, deformities or asymmetry

2. Lightly palpate the chest to assess for any signs of tenderness, pain or masses

3. To assess for chest expansion place thumbs along each costal margin at about the 5th/6th rib with fingers fanned out towards the lateral chest. Ask the patient to take a deep breath in

4. To assess for tactile fremitus place the edge of your palm and little finger on the patient's chest and ask the patient to say 99

5. Percuss the chest to assess for a normal resonant lung and identifying any abnormalities

6. Auscultate the lung using the bell of the stethoscope for the apex of the lung: above the clavicle and the diaphragm of the stethoscope for the rest of the chest to assess for vesicular breath sounds and any adventitious sounds

7. Document the full procedures and findings in the patients records

8. Report any abnormal findings to the Doctor

9. Explain the findings to the patient and discuss plan of care

10. Decontaminate hands according to correct hand hygiene techniques and clean the stethoscope according to manufacturer's guidelines

References
Bickley, L. Szilagyi, P. Hoffman, R. (2017). *Bates Guide to Physical Examination and History Taking.* 12th edn. Philadelphia: Lipincott Williams & Wilkins.
Dougherty, L. & Lister, S. (2015). The Royal Marsden Hospital Manual of Clinical Nursing Procedures. 9th Ed. Wiley Blackwell Pub: Chichester.

27. Cardiovascular Examination Guidelines

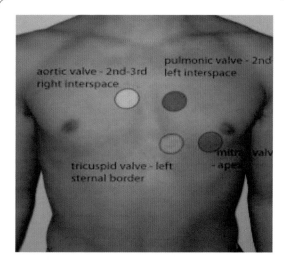

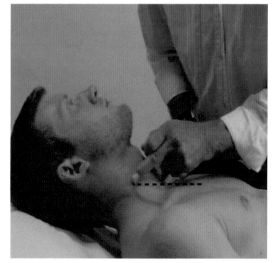

Equipment

- Stethoscope
- Examination couch
- Pen torch
- Tongue depressor
- Ruler

Procedure

1. Explain the procedure to the patient and gain informed consent

2. Ask the patient to empty their bladder as a full bladder will interfere with the examination

3. Make sure the patient is comfortable and ideally in the supine position, with their head at a 30 - 45 degree angle and arms by their sides

4. Ensure privacy and ask the patient to remove garments above the waist. Access to the legs will also be required

5. Decontaminate hands according to correct hand hygiene techniques

General inspection

6. Look at the patient's skin and nails. Feel the temperature, texture and turgor of the skin

7. To assess for capillary refill press the patient's fingernail firmly for 5 seconds between your finger and thumb and then let go. Count how many seconds it takes for the colour to return to the nail

8. Look at the patients eyes, to assess for any abnormalities and signs of hypercholesterolaemia and anaemia

9. Look at and in the patients mouth to check for any abnormalities, sores, infection, central cyanosis

10. To assess jugular venous pressure ask the patient to turn their head to the left, use tangential lighting and locate the highest pulsation point of the internal jugular vein. Place a ruler vertically from the sternal angle, then place a tongue depressor placed horizontally to make a right angle from the pulsation to the ruler. The jugular venous pressure is measured in centimetres and the measurement is where the tongue depressor meets the ruler

11. Inspect the precordium to assess for scars, deformities, heaves, lifts and the apical impulse

12. Inspect the legs to assess for signs of venous disease and ischaemic changes

Palpation

13. Palpate the pulses to assess cardiac output

14. Palpate the chest to assess for tenderness, heaves, lifts and thrills

15. To assess for apical impulse palpate with the fingertips the 5th intercostal space midclavicular line

Auscultation

16. Listen with the bell of the stethoscope to the carotid pulse to assess for bruits

17. Auscultate at the aortic, pulmonary, tricuspid and mitral valves with the diaphragm of the stethoscope to assess S1 and S2

18. Auscultate at the aortic, pulmonary, tricuspid and mitral valves with the bell of the stethoscope to assess S3 and S4 and murmurs

19. Ask the patient to roll partially onto their left side and listen with the bell of the stethoscope to the apical impulse to assess for a mitral murmur

20. Ask the patient to sit up and lean forward, exhale completely and hold their breath. Listen with the diaphragm of the stethoscope to the apical impulse and along the left sternal border to assess for an aortic murmur and pericardial friction rubs

21. Ask the patient to sit up and listen to the lung bases with the diaphragm of the stethoscope to assess for lung congestion that can be caused by heart failure

22. Document and record all findings in the patients notes

23. Report any abnormal findings to the doctor

24. Explain the findings to the patient and discuss plan of care

25. Decontaminate hands according to correct hand hygiene techniques and clean any equipment used according to manufacturer's guidelines

References

Bickley, L. Szilagyi, P. Hoffman, R. (2017). *Bates Guide to Physical Examination and History Taking.* 12th edn. Philadelphia: Lipincott Williams & Wilkins.

Dougherty, L. & Lister, S. (2015). The Royal Marsden Hospital Manual of Clinical Nursing Procedures. 9th Ed. Wiley Blackwell Pub: Chichester. Dougherty, L. & Lister, S. (2015). The Royal Marsden Hospital Manual of Clinical Nursing Procedures. 9th Ed. Wiley Blackwell Pub: Chichester.

28. Abdominal Examination Guidelines

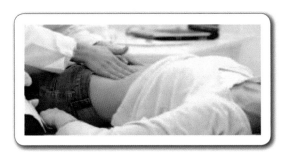

Equipment

- Stethoscope
- Examination couch
- Pen torch
- Tongue depressor

Procedure

1. Explain the procedure to the patient and gain informed consent

2. Ask the patient to empty their bladder as a full bladder will interfere with the examination

3. Make sure the patient is comfortable and ideally in the supine position, with their head at a 30 - 45 degree angle and arms by their side

4. Ensure privacy and expose from nipple to pubis, maintaining dignity at all times

5. Decontaminate hands according to correct hand hygiene techniques

General inspection

6. Look at the patient's skin and nails. Feel the temperature, texture and turgor of the skin. Abnormalities of the skin and nails can be an indication of a variety of different conditions, e.g. bowel disease, malnutrition, liver disease, dehydration and anaemia

7. To assess for liver flaps (signs of liver and or renal failure) ask the patient to extend their arms, flex their wrists and part their fingers. Ask them to stay in this position for 15 seconds

8. Look at the patients eyes to assess for any abnormalities and signs of jaundice, example hyper - cholesterolaemia and anaemia

9. Look at the patients nose to assess for signs of telangiectasia which can indicate liver disease

10. Look at and in the patients mouth to check for any abnormalities, sores, infection and malnutrition

11. Smell the patients breath to assess for signs of fetor, A sweet smelling breath can be a sign of ketoacidosis

12. Ask the patient to shrug their shoulders and lightly palpate, using the finger tips, directly above the clavicle, to assess for a raised supraclavicular lymph node which can indicate gastrointestinal malignancy

13. Move to the foot of the bed to inspect the abdomen

14. Observe the contour of the abdomen and position of the umbilicus to assess for asymmetry or distension, peristalsis and or pulsation

15. Move to the side of the bed and observe the contour of the abdomen

16. Look at the patients skin to observe for signs of spider naevi, striae, scars, caput medusa, bruising and rashes

17. Auscultation

18. Using the diaphragm of the stethoscope, listen in all four quadrants for 1 minute to assess for bowel sounds

19. Using the bell of the stethoscope, listen over the aortic, renal, iliac and femoral arteries to assess for bruits

Percussion

20. Percuss in 9 areas of the abdomen to listen for a normal distribution of tympany and dullness

21. Percuss for liver span to assess the size and location of the liver. Percuss upwards starting in the right lower quadrant, midclavicular line. Stop when you hear the dullness of the liver. Next percuss down, starting from the nipple line, midclavicular: stop when the sound changes from the resonant lung to the dull liver. Measure between these two points

22. While not routinely done the above technique can be employed to percuss the spleen, bladder and kidneys especially if organomegaly is suspected

Palpation

23. Lightly palpate the abdomen using one hand to assess for tenderness, rebound tenderness, superficial organs or masses. Look at the patients face at all times to make sure they are not in pain

24. Deeply palpate the abdomen to assess organs and deeper masses

25. To assess for hepatomegaly and gallbladder tenderness (known as Murphy's sign) palpate for the liver by placing the left hand in the small of the patients back and the right in the right lower quadrant pointing towards the upper left quadrant. Ask the patient to take a deep breath and palpate up. If nothing is felt, move up towards the liver and repeat until the ribcage is reached

26. To assess for splenomegaly, palpate for the spleen. Ask the patient to tip slightly onto their right side. Start from the umbilicus region and use the technique mentioned above moving towards the spleen

27. To assess for kidney enlargement, palpate for the kidneys. (If the kidney is normal it is not usually palpable). Palpate each kidney separately. For the right kidney, stand on the right side of the patient, place the left hand just below the 12th rib and lift up. Place the other hand on the right upper quadrant of the abdomen. Ask the patient to take a deep breath and press the right hand deeply into the abdomen, trying to feel the kidney between the hands. Repeat for the left side.

28. Lightly palpate each costovertebral angle for tenderness; if none is felt place one hand flat over the costovertebral angle and strike the hand firmly with the other fist. Pain can indicate pyelonephritis

29. Document and record all findings in the patients notes

30. Report any abnormal findings to the doctor

31. Explain the findings to the patient and discuss plan of care

32. Decontaminate hands using correct hand hygiene techniques and clean any equipment used according to manufacturer's instructions

References

Bickley, L. Szilagyi, P. Hoffman, R. (2017). *Bates Guide to Physical Examination and History Taking.* 12th edn. Philadelphia: Lipincott Williams & Wilkins.

Dougherty, L. & Lister, S. (2015). The Royal Marsden Hospital Manual of Clinical Nursing Procedures. 9th Ed. Wiley Blackwell Pub: Chichester.Dougherty, L. & Lister, S. (2015). The Royal Marsden Hospital Manual of Clinical Nursing Procedures. 9th Ed. Wiley Blackwell Pub: Chichester.

29. Cervical Screening Guidelines

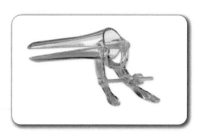

Equipment

- Examination couch
- A height - adjustable couch
- Adjustable light source
- Adequate drapes and privacy
- A disposable sheet, pillow and blanket cover such as couch roll should be used
- Speculums (plastic disposable is preferable) in different sizes. At least three different sizes of bivalve vaginal speculum should be available: small, medium, and large. A very small speculum (virgin speculum) and a long - bladed narrow speculum may occasionally be needed
- Steriliser if using reusable specula. A systematic and documented system must be in place that follows manufacturers' guidelines if reusable specula are used. Disposable specula are preferable
- Water based lubricant (if required). A soluble lubricant such as KY Jelly should be used carefully if the vagina is very dry. Care must be taken to use only a little on the shaft and avoid use at the tip of the speculum
- The sampling tool is the Cervex Brush®
- The single test for smear tests taken in Ireland is liquid based cytology (LBC)
- The transport medium is a liquid - filled vial. Liquid - Based Cytology (LBC) vial
- LBC transport boxes
- Additional testing equipment if required (e.g. STI, HPV). Chlamydia and charcoal swabs available for the evaluation of infectious discharge
- Disposable Gloves. Vinyl or latex disposable gloves are recommended
- Tissues
- Cervical Cytology request forms
- Waste disposal bags Clinical waste needs to be disposed of with care, especially used disposable specula and samplers

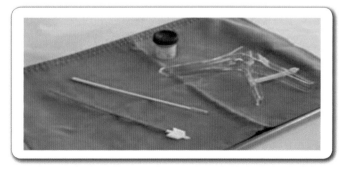

Procedure

1. An appropriate history - taking and consultation with the woman is undertaken and any individual special requirements should be accommodated. History taking questions should include: Any abnormal bleeding: Post - coital bleeding (PCB):Inter - menstrual bleeding (IMB): Post - menopausal bleeding (PMB): Any unusual vaginal discharge: Any pain or discomfort with sexual intercourse

2. Women having a cervical smear test taken should be counselled before, during and after the procedure. The woman's understanding of the test and her concerns about its implications must be fully addressed. Clear language should be used. It is important to check with the woman that she understands all the information provided

3. It should be emphasised that the smear test is not a test for cancer. It is a screening test only

4. Gain informed consent. Consent to have the smear test taken is implicit when the woman allows the test to occur. However, this should only occur after a full explanation. Informed consent includes the giving of all necessary information by the smear taker; this includes the benefits and limitations of cervical screening

5. Offer the option of a chaperone. The Irish Medical Council guidelines for doctor's states that any intimate examination should be accompanied by an explanation and the patient, irrespective of age or gender, should be offered a chaperone. If the woman refuses a chaperone, record in the clinical notes that a chaperone was offered and declined

6. Before the test ensure that all the necessary supplies and equipment are checked and in date and set up on a trolley

7. The smear taker's hands must be washed before and after any procedure that involves close contact with the patient

8. The woman should be allowed an opportunity to empty her bladder

9. Ask the woman to undress from the waist down and to lie on the couch. The woman may be more comfortable leaving a skirt on but removal of trousers is needed to allow for adequate exposure and good lighting of the perineum

10. Ensure that privacy is maintained by using a couch roll as a cover rather than a blanket or sheet where infection control could be compromised. The position of the woman is important and the time spent ensuring she is in the correct position will make finding the cervix easier

11. Smear tests can be taken in the dorsal position or in the left lateral position. The dorsal position allows for better communication and observation of the woman and is the most common position to take a smear test. In the dorsal position, the woman lies with the buttocks towards the light source, soles of feet together, knees bent and legs lax but wide open. If there is difficulty when smear taking, it can be effective to reposition the woman and for her to place her fists under her buttocks. Some women may be used to having smear tests taken in the left lateral position and may put themselves in that position. The left lateral position may be better for visualising the cervix if the uterus is acutely anteverted or retroverted

12. It is important to help the woman to relax. For some women, explanation of the various steps in the procedure helps them to relax

13. A confident, unrushed approach is helpful and good practice recommends that the first touch to the woman should be on her arm or leg by way of reassurance

Location and visualising the cervix

14. Ensure privacy, comfort and adequate lighting before beginning the procedure

15. Ensure the patient is comfortable with legs correctly positioned on the bed/couch

16. Decontaminate hands using correct hand hygiene techniques and wear disposable gloves

17. Choose a speculum. A tray or trolley with the appropriate equipment and full range of specula should be close at hand. When choosing a speculum, the age, parity and size of the woman should be taken into consideration. When using a disposable speculum, the package should not be opened until ready for use. When using reusable specula, a range of sizes should be available and in a sterile state

Insertion of the speculum

18. The largest size speculum that can be comfortably inserted should be chosen. The appropriate size will be helpful in holding back the vaginal walls. A long speculum is usually required for tall women. It can also be useful when the cervix is in a posterior position. In obese women, or women with a lax vagina, sheathing the speculum with the finger of a large surgical glove, having cut the tip of the finger (this forms a cylinder) may prevent the vaginal walls from obscuring the cervix

19. The smear taker should check the temperature of the speculum and adjust to body temperature. This, however, is not necessary with disposable plastic specula which are preferred and recommended for use

20. After inspection of the vulva, the labia should be separated and the speculum inserted gently but firmly along the axis of the introitus, with the speculum pointing downwards and backwards. When the speculum is half way up the vagina, it should be rotated gently through 90 degrees

21. It is important to angle the speculum towards the patient's coccyx and not to open the speculum until it is fully inserted. Opening and closing the speculum and changing the angle of insertion should bring the cervix into view. A common error is failure to insert the speculum far enough into the vagina

22. It is helpful to allow a little time after passing the speculum to allow the woman to relax. Lubrication of the speculum is usually not necessary but if the vagina is very dry, a little water or a small amount of soluble lubricant, such as KY Jelly, can be applied

23. Having visualised the entire cervix and identified the squamocolumnar junction, the long central bristles of the Cervex - Brush® are inserted into the external cervical os, ensuring good contact is made

24. Sweep the brush around the whole Transformation Zone including the margins. It is important that the sample is taken with care so that the Cervex - Brush® is firmly rotated to a full 360 degrees, five times in a clockwise direction. This should be done using 'pencil' pressure by rolling the stem between the thumb and the forefinger, ensuring that the lateral bristles bend against the ectocervix and maintain good contact throughout

25. Copious cervical mucous can be removed before taking the smear test by gently twisting the other end of the Cervex Brush® in the mucous, avoiding contact with the cervix, and then 'lifting' the mucous off the cervix

26. Once the sample is taken withdraw the speculum gently with the blades apart until the cervix is no longer within the blades. Allow the speculum to close and continue to withdraw without pinching the vaginal walls

27. Provide the woman with tissues to clean/wipe the vaginal area after the smear

Preparation of sample for the laboratory

28. The cells need to be transferred directly into the liquid and this is done immediately with vigorous 'mash and bash' action to ensure maximum yield. It is recommended that the bristles of the brush are pushed vigorously against the bottom of the specimen vial ten times, ensuring that the bristles are pushed apart. It should look distorted when the sample has been prepared

29. The Cervex - Brush® should then be rinsed by rotating the shaft of the brush between the finger and thumb and should be inspected for any residual material. Any remains should be removed by passing the brush over the edge of the vial but do not stand Cervex - Brush® in liquid at any time

30. The cap should be tightened, but not over - tightened, so that the line on the cap passes the torque line on the vial. The vial can be shaken if any material has been placed on the edge of the vial. The Cervex - Brush®/ sampler may then be discarded with the clinical waste

Submitting samples to the laboratory.

31. The Cervical Cytology Form is designed to ensure that the right woman gets the right result. Complete, current and accurate demographic information is necessary and all information recorded in the Cervical Cytology Form must be legible

32. Fill in the form at the time of smear taking in the presence of the woman to check the accuracy of personal details

33. There is a minimum data set of information required when completing the Cervical Cytology form, which helps to match the right results to the right woman. The Cervical Check minimum dataset is as follows: Date of birth (DOB): Forename: Surname at birth: Mother's maiden name: Personal Public Service Number (PPS No): Middle names: Surname: Address and Phone number

34. Relevant clinical detail required (Boxes to tick on Cervical Cytology Form) are: Date of Cervical Screening: Cervix visualised: LMP: HRT: Pregnant: Post colposcopy smear: IUCD: Post - menopausal. This information helps the cytologist to make an accurate recommendation when viewing cells at cytology.

35. Describe what is seen at the time of smear taking on the referral form. Discharge, warts, polyps may be of relevance to the cytologist and should be recorded in the clinical findings box

36. Details of the woman's previous two smear test results if available (whether normal or abnormal) and information and details of any abnormal smear tests in the past (especially in the last 10 years) must be recorded on the form

37. Information relating to any previous colposcopy treatment of the cervix should be recorded where available, including year of treatment and discharge recommendations

38. The address on the Cervical Cytology Form is the address to which all letters and contacts with the woman are directed. Eligible women must be normally resident and have a postal address in the Republic of Ireland

39. The vials can be left at room temperature and should not be placed in a fridge and must be posted within five working days, even if the transport box is not full. It is however recommended that the samples are posted to the laboratory on the day of the test. Each vial reaching the laboratory must be accompanied by a corresponding Cervical Cytology Form. Label the vial with a pen. The laboratory will reject the sample if it cannot match the details on the form to the details on the sample

40. Marked vials and forms must be packaged in the transport containers provided

41. Boxes are reusable and should not be written on. It is advisable to log the day of posting the smear test and one 'bar code' label should be retained when posting to allow for tracing in the event that a package is lost in transit

42. To facilitate the delivery of a result to a woman within four weeks it is important to dispatch the sample promptly. It is the responsibility of the Smear taker (not the woman) to dispatch/post samples

Quick guide summary

1. Write identification details on the Cervical Cytology Form and the liquid base vial

2. Choose the appropriate speculum for the woman

3. Identify and visualise the cervix

4. Take a sample from the entire squamocolumnar junction

5. Rinse the cells immediately into the vial and cap

6. Put into a suitable transport container

7. Record details of the smear test on the Cervical Cytology Form and in the woman's clinical notes

8. Enter the smear test in a practice tracking system, manual or electronic

9. Post promptly to the laboratory to minimise turnaround time

Adapted from: Cervical Check (2011) Guide for smear takers (2nd Edn). The National Cancer Screening Service. Ireland

Important Note

The HPV Screening Test (approved by HIQA, May 2017) a more accurate cervical screening service is expected to be introduced next year (2019) to replace the current screening service. Please refer to new Government guidelines and publications when available.

30. Vaginal Swab Guidelines

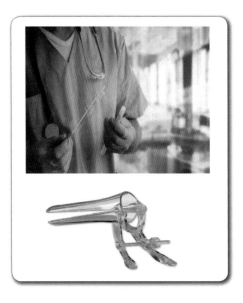

Equipment

- Non sterile gloves
- Apron
- Sterile swabs (bacterial or viral) with transport medium
- Microbiology request forms
- Light source
- Sterile speculum

Procedure

1. Explain the procedure to the patient and gain informed consent
2. Set up the equipment on a trolley
3. Position patient on the couch bed with knees bent and legs apart. Adjust the light
4. Decontaminate hands using correct hand hygiene techniques
5. Apply apron and gloves
6. Remove appropriate swab (s) (Bacterial/Viral) from outer packaging
7. For low vaginal swab, insert the swab into the lower part of the vagina and rotate gently but firmly
8. For high vaginal swab, moisten the speculum with warm water and insert into the vagina to separate the vaginal walls. Wipe away any excess cervical mucus with a cotton swab. Using a sterile swab sample as high as possible in the vaginal vault. Remove speculum and wipe the vaginal/ vulval area with a tissue
9. Allow patient to resume a comfortable position
10. Remove cap from the transport tube
11. Carefully place swab into the transport tube, ensuring it is fully immersed in the transport medium. Ensure cap is secure. Label swab with full identifying details
12. Remove gloves and apron and wash/ decontaminate hands
13. Complete the microbiology request form with patient details, including relevant information such as exact site, nature of specimen and investigation required. Arrange delivery to the laboratory
14. Document the procedure in the patients notes

31. Managing Diabetic Patients in General Practice Guidelines

Practice Nurse Responsibilities

- Provide regular routine care in the practice to patients with diabetes
- Maintain practice diabetes register
- Set targets with patients
- Provide patient education: Diet/lifestyle/exercise etc.
- Carry out initial and annual foot assessment per national model
- Refer patients to community diabetes nurse specialist
- Refer patients for retinal screening, dietetics and podiatry

The Role of the Integrated Care Diabetes Nurse Specialist

The Integrated Care Diabetes Nurse Specialist (DNS) is the health care professional who ensures successful integration of patient care between primary and secondary care.

The nurse specialist works 80% in primary care and 20% in secondary care.

The CNS (Diabetes - Integrated Care) will have a clinical reporting relationship with the GP whose patients they are seeing in primary care and with the Consultant Endocrinologist in secondary care.

The Integrated Care Diabetes Nurse Specialist will;

- See individual patients referred by the GP/PN
- Provide training and support to PN's within the GP practice to set up and deliver integrated care
- Deliver educational programmes in conjunction with the local nursing education units, for example the HETAC Certificate in Diabetes, along with annual multidisciplinary master classes
- Carry out research and audit, including using audit data to influence the delivery of integrated care at practice level

References

Department of Health and Children (2016). Irish College of General Practitioners– A Practical Guide to Integrated Type 2 Diabetes Care. DOH: Dublin

32. Managing Diabetic Patients in General Practice Guidelines

Collect Demographic details	Yes	No
Patient name/ address/DOB/gender/ ethnicity		
Type of Diabetes - Uncomplicated Type 2 / Complicated Type 2/ Other		
Smoker		
Alcohol		

Dianosis of Diabetes	Yes	No
Date (year) of Diagnosis		
Osmotic symptoms		
Random plasma glucose		
Fasting plasma glucose		
2hour OGTT		
Fasting plasma glucose		
HbA1C		
Current medications & compliance history		
Family History of Diabetes		
Gestational Diabetes		

Past Medical History:		Yes	No
	Coronary Artery Disease		
	MI		
	CVA		
	TIA		
	PAD		
	Erectile dysfuncti on		
	Thyroid disease		
	Other		

Examination		Yes	No
Weight/Height - Calculate BMI			
Blood Pressure			
Foot examination (as per National Model of Foot - Care)	Foot pulses		
	10gm monofilament		
	Vibration sensation		
Waist circumference			

Investigation	Yes	No
HbA1c		
Fasting Lipid Profile		
Full Blood Count		
Renal Function - Serum Creatinine, Urine Albumin Creatinine Ratio (ACR), eGFR		
Thyroid Function Tests		
Liver Function Tests		
Ferritin – serum iron/ transferrin saturation (if ferritin raised)		
12 lead ECG		

Referral	Yes	No
Practice nurse education		
Structured education programme		
Exercise advice		
Dietitian*		
Podiatry		
Retinal screening		
Self Monitoring Blood glucose		
Clinical Nurse Specialist		
Add patient to practice register and give follow - up appointment		
Nominate Secondary Centre if appropriate		

*: If not suitable for group structured education programme at time of diagnosis refer for individual session with dietitian

33. Regular Review

Regular review is needed every four months or more frequently during efforts to bring risk factors under control. The aim of regular review is prevention, early detection and management of complications

Regular review includes the following elements		Yes	No
Medications			
Hypoglycaemia/hyperglycemia			
Smoking Status			
Dietary Habits			
Physical activity			
Assess injection sites if on insulin			
Recent life - events / new symptoms			
Other medical conditions and therapy affecting diabetes, psychological, lifestyle and social aspects			
Examination		Yes	No
Weight/Height – calculate BMI			
Blood pressure			
Foot examination as per National Model of Foot care	Foot pulse		
	10gm monofilament		
	Vibration sensation		
Investigations		Yes	No
HbA1c			
Recheck Lipids if raised at first or preceding review			
Urinalysis and ACR, calculate eGFR (if raised at first or preceding review)			
Blood pressure			
Referral follow - up		Yes	No
Practice nurse education			
Structured education programme			
Retinal screening			
Podiatry			
Exercise advice			
Dietitian			
Podiatry			
Smoking Cessation			
Self management Blood Glucose Monitoring			
Pre - conceptual advice			

References
Department of Health and Children (2016). Irish College of General Practitioners– A Practical Guide to Integrated Type 2 Diabetes Care. DOH: Dublin.

34. Annual Review Assessment

Topics to be covered with patient
What is Diabetes
Dietary Management
Eye and Foot Care
Behaviour modification
Motivation Strategies
Complications
Aims of Diabetes Care
Why self - monitoring may be needed
Key self - care issues to be covered with patient
Medications: Uses and Side - Effects
Self - Monitoring, if indicated
Hypoglycaemia
Allowances, Entitlements
Hyperglycaemia
Membership of Diabetes Ireland
Sick - Days
Additional issues as appropriate for specific patient
Lifestyle: smoking, alcohol, exercise,
Employment, Insurance, Driving issues weight control
New Symptoms:
Cardiovascular Status: Hypertension,
Nocturia: frequency
Hyperlipidaemia, Micro - albuminuria
Dry mouth
Managing Insulin
Chest pain: Sensation, Dyspepsia
Travel Advice
Visual disturbance
Encouraging Self - care
Foot problems
Discussion with Carers
Impotence
Family Planning or Pre - Conception
Advice

Symptoms
Ischaemic heart disease, peripheral vascular disease - neuropathy, erectile dysfunction. All patients with symptoms that might reflect vascular disease, particularly ischaemic heart disease, should be investigated

Feet
Footwear, deformity/joint rigidity, poor skin condition, ischaemia, ulceration, absent pulses, sensory impairment

Eyes
Visual acuity and retinal review by ophthalmologist/retinal screening programme

Kidney
Renal damage, albumin excretion, serum creatinine and eGFR

Arterial risk
Blood glucose, blood pressure, blood lipids, smoking status, ECG

Attendances
Podiatry/dietitian/other as indicated

Foot Assessment and Classification Protocol

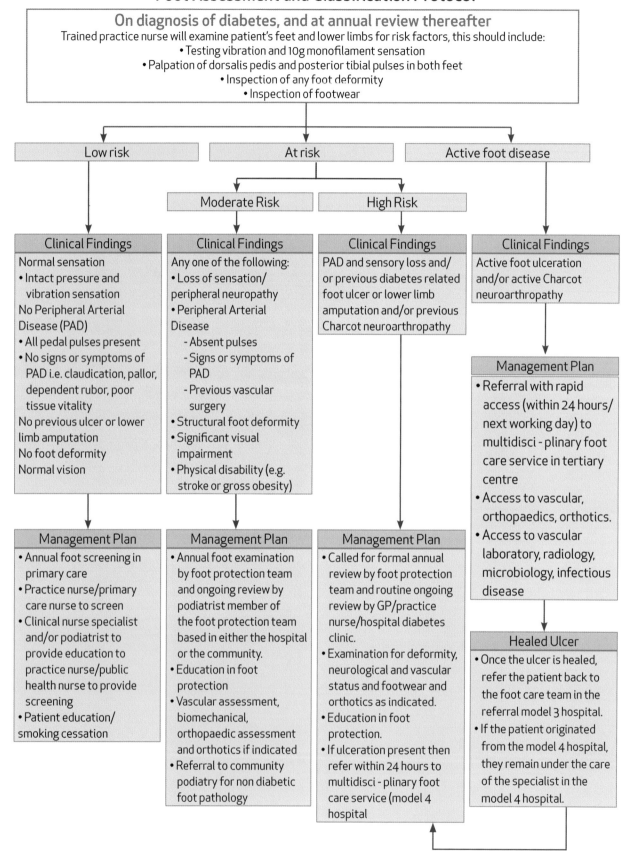

On diagnosis of diabetes, and at annual review thereafter

Trained practice nurse will examine patient's feet and lower limbs for risk factors, this should include:
- Testing vibration and 10g monofilament sensation
- Palpation of dorsalis pedis and posterior tibial pulses in both feet
- Inspection of any foot deformity
- Inspection of footwear

Low risk	At risk	Active foot disease

	Moderate Risk	High Risk	

Clinical Findings

Normal sensation
- Intact pressure and vibration sensation

No Peripheral Arterial Disease (PAD)
- All pedal pulses present
- No signs or symptoms of PAD i.e. claudication, pallor, dependent rubor, poor tissue vitality

No previous ulcer or lower limb amputation

No foot deformity

Normal vision

Clinical Findings

Any one of the following:
- Loss of sensation/ peripheral neuropathy
- Peripheral Arterial Disease
  - Absent pulses
  - Signs or symptoms of PAD
  - Previous vascular surgery
- Structural foot deformity
- Significant visual impairment
- Physical disability (e.g. stroke or gross obesity)

Clinical Findings

PAD and sensory loss and/ or previous diabetes related foot ulcer or lower limb amputation and/or previous Charcot neuroarthropathy

Clinical Findings

Active foot ulceration and/or active Charcot neuroarthropathy

Management Plan
- Referral with rapid access (within 24 hours/ next working day) to multidisci - plinary foot care service in tertiary centre
- Access to vascular, orthopaedics, orthotics.
- Access to vascular laboratory, radiology, microbiology, infectious disease

Management Plan
- Annual foot screening in primary care
- Practice nurse/primary care nurse to screen
- Clinical nurse specialist and/or podiatrist to provide education to practice nurse/public health nurse to provide screening
- Patient education/ smoking cessation

Management Plan
- Annual foot examination by foot protection team and ongoing review by podiatrist member of the foot protection team based in either the hospital or the community.
- Education in foot protection
- Vascular assessment, biomechanical, orthopaedic assessment and orthotics if indicated
- Referral to community podiatry for non diabetic foot pathology

Management Plan
- Called for formal annual review by foot protection team and routine ongoing review by GP/practice nurse/hospital diabetes clinic.
- Examination for deformity, neurological and vascular status and footwear and orthotics as indicated.
- Education in foot protection.
- If ulceration present then refer within 24 hours to multidisci - plinary foot care service (model 4 hospital

Healed Ulcer
- Once the ulcer is healed, refer the patient back to the foot care team in the referral model 3 hospital.
- If the patient originated from the model 4 hospital, they remain under the care of the specialist in the model 4 hospital.

Source: HSE Model of Care for the Diabetic Foot

Diabetes foot screening tool

Patient Name: ....

Patient Address: ....

....

....

....

....

DOB: ....

Phone No: ....

....

❒ Medical card   ❒ Long term illness card   ❒ neither

Diabetes: ❒ Type 1   ❒ Type 2

Date of latest HbA1c ....: IFCC .... mmol/L

Medication: ....

....

....

History of:
❒ retinopathy   ❒ nephropathy   ❒ MI   ❒ CVA

Smoker: ❒ Yes   ❒ No

Anticoagulant Therapy: ❒ Yes   ❒ No

GP Name: ....

GP Address..

....

....

Lower Limb Vascular Assessment

Right Foot

Left Foot

PT pulse: ❒ Present ❒ Absent	DP pulse: ❒ Present ❒ Absent	PT pulse: ❒ Present ❒ Absent	DP pulse: ❒ Present ❒ Absent
Int. Claudication: ❒ Yes ❒ No	Rest Pain: ❒ Yes ❒ No	Int. Claudication: ❒ Yes ❒ No	Rest Pain: ❒ Yes ❒ No
Oedema: ❒ Yes ❒ No		Oedema: ❒ Yes ❒ No	
Diabetes Related Amputation	❒ Yes ❒ No if Yes: ❒ BKA ❒ AKA ❒ TMA ❒ Digital	Diabetes Related Amputation	❒ Yes ❒ No if Yes: ❒ BKA ❒ AKA ❒ TMA ❒ Digital

Peripheral Sensory Assessment

Right Foot

Left Foot

Vibration Sensation (tuning fork 128HZ): ❒ Present ❒ Absent	Vibration Sensation (tuning fork 128HZ): ❒ Present ❒ Absent

Diabetes foot screening tool

10g Monofilament: tick circle site if present, cross if **not**

Foot Wounds:

Right Foot			Left Foot:		
Foot Ulcer	☐ Yes	☐ No	Foot Ulcer	☐ Yes	☐ No
Previous Foot Ulcer	☐ Yes	☐ No	Previous Foot Ulcer	☐ Yes	☐ No

Foot Deformity:

Right Foot			Left Foot:		
Bunion	☐ Yes	☐ No	Bunion	☐ Yes	☐ No
Claw Toes	☐ Yes	☐ No	Claw Toes	☐ Yes	☐ No

Skin and Nail Condition:

Right Foot			Left Foot:		
Skin dry	☐ Yes	☐ No	Skin dry	☐ Yes	☐ No
Plantar Callous	☐ Yes	☐ No	Plantar Callous	☐ Yes	☐ No
Ingrowing Nail(s)	☐ Yes	☐ No	Ingrowing Nail(s)	☐ Yes	☐ No
Thickened Nail(s)	☐ Yes	☐ No	Thickened Nail(s)	☐ Yes	☐ No

Footwear Assessment:

Foot Wear: Good Fit (Not too loose/too tight)	☐ Yes	☐ No
Foot Wear: Good Shape (Square box toe – not pointed)	☐ Yes	☐ No
Foot Wear: Lace/Velcro (Slip on not appropriate)	☐ Yes	☐ No

Risk Level:

☐ Low Risk	☐ Mod Risk	☐ High Risk	☐ Active Foot Disease
Arrange Annual Review	Refer to Podiatry	Refer to Podiatry	Refer to Multidisciplinary Foot Care Service

Signature: ....

Job Position: ....

Printed Name: ....

Date: ....

35. New: Type 1 Diabetes (Adult) Guidelines (DOH, 2018)

The UK's National Institute for Health and Care Excellence (NICE) provides evidence - based guidance and advice to improve health and social care. In 2017 an agreement was reached between NICE and the National Patient Safety Office's Clinical Effectiveness Unit, on behalf of the NCEC to work together on the contextualisation of NICE's clinical guideline, (NG17) Type 1 diabetes in adults: diagnosis and management (2015).

This National Clinical Guideline applies to adults (aged 18 years and older) with type 1 diabetes in Ireland. It does not apply to children living with type 1 diabetes, adults living with type 2 diabetes or individuals living with monogenic (or other rarer forms of) diabetes. The National Clinical Guideline is relevant to all healthcare professionals working in healthcare settings delivering care to people living with type 1 diabetes.

The National Clinical Guideline Summary Main Recommendations
Education and information
- Offer all adults with type 1 diabetes a structured education programme of proven benefit, for example the DAFNE (dose - adjustment for normal eating) programme. Offer this programme 6–12 months after diagnosis

Blood glucose management
- Support adults with type 1 diabetes to aim for a target HbA1c level of 48 mmol/mol (6.5%) or lower, to minimise the risk of long - term vascular complications
- Agree an individualised HbA1c target with each adult with type 1 diabetes, taking into account factors such as the person's daily activities, aspirations, likelihood of complications, comorbidities, occupation and history of hypoglycaemia
- Support adults with type 1 diabetes to test at least 4 times a day, and up to 10 times a day if any of the following apply:
    - the desired target for blood glucose control, measured by HbA1c level is not achieved
    - the frequency of hypoglycaemic episodes increases
    - there is a legal requirement to do so, such as before driving, in line with the Road Safety Authority (RSA) (2014) Sláinte agus Tiomáint Medical Fitness to Drive Guidelines
    - during periods of illness
    - before, during and after vigorous physical activity

- when planning pregnancy, during pregnancy and while breastfeeding, see the HSE (2010) Guidelines for the Management of Pre - gestational and Gestational Diabetes Mellitus and the NICE (2015) Guideline Diabetes in pregnancy: management from preconception to the postnatal period (NG3)
    - if there is a need to know blood glucose levels more than 4 times a day for other reasons (for example, impaired awareness of hypoglycaemia, high - risk activities)
- Advise adults with type 1 diabetes to aim for: a fasting plasma glucose level of 5–7 mmol/litre on waking and a plasma glucose level of 4–7 mmol/litre before meals at other times of the day

Insulin therapy

- Offer multiple daily injection basal–bolus insulin regimens, rather than twice - daily mixed insulin regimens, as the insulin injection regimen of choice for all adults with type 1 diabetes. Provide the person with guidance on using multiple daily injection basal - bolus insulin regimens

Awareness and management of hypoglycaemia

- Assess awareness of hypoglycaemia in adults with type 1 diabetes at each annual review

Care of adults with type 1 diabetes in hospital

- Enable adults with type 1 diabetes who are hospital inpatients to self - administer subcutaneous insulin if they are willing and able and it is safe to do so

Key priorities for implementation

- To provide access to high quality structured patient education programmes for eligible adults with type 1 diabetes in Ireland 6 – 12 months after diagnosis or at another appropriate time.
- Measure HbA1c levels every 3–6 months in adults with type 1 diabetes. To facilitate implementation provide access to a minimum of 2 consultations with a diabetes healthcare provider per year for all adults with type 1

Refer to the full document and Guidelines at:
Department of Health (2018). Adult type 1 diabetes mellitus (NCEC National Clinical Guideline No. 17). DOH: Dublin. Available at: http://health.gov.ie/national - patient - safety - office/ncec.

36. Ear Irrigation Guidelines

Equipment

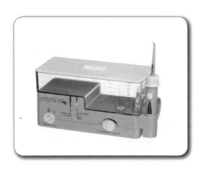

- Otoscope
- Electronic ear irrigator (example Pro - pulse)
- Disposable ear probe / tip applicator
- Tap water at 37o
- Receiver/ trough
- Tissues and receivers for dirty swabs and instruments
- Disposable waterproof cape and paper towels
- Disposable apron and gloves

Irrigation should NOT be carried out when

- The patient has previously experienced complications following this procedure in the past
- There is a history of a middle ear infection in the last six weeks
- The patient has undergone ANY form of ear surgery (apart from grommets that have extruded at least 18 months previously and the patient has been discharged from the ENT Department)
- The patient has a perforation or there is a history of a mucous discharge in the last year
- The patient has a cleft palate (repaired or not)
- There is evidence of acute otitis externa with pain and tenderness of the pinna

Precautions

- Tinnitus
- Healed Perforation Dizziness

Procedure

1. Explain the procedure to the patient and obtain informed consent
2. Decontaminate hands and apply non - sterile gloves and apron
3. Examine both ears by first inspecting the pinna and adjacent scalp.

4. Check for previous surgery incision scars or skin defects, then inspect the EAM with the otoscope

5. Check whether the patient has had his/her ears irrigated previously, or if there are any contra - indications why irrigation should not be performed

6. Check that the patient is seated correctly and comfortably

7. Place the protective cape and paper towel on the patient's shoulder and under the ear to be irrigated. Ask the patient to hold the receiver under the same ear

8. Check that the temperature of the water is approximately 37°C and fill the reservoir of the irrigator. Set the pressure at minimum

9. Connect a new ear probe jet tip applicator to the tubing of the machine with a firm 'push/twist' action. Push until a "click" is felt

10. Switch on the machine for 10 - 20 seconds in order to circulate the water through the system and eliminate any trapped air or cold water. This offers the opportunity for the patient to become accustomed to the noise of the machine

11. Twist the jet tip/ ear probe so that the water can be aimed along the posterior wall of the EAM (towards the back of the patient's head)

12. Gently pull the pinna upwards and outwards to straighten the EAM

13. Explain to the patient that you are about to start irrigating and that the procedure will be stopped immediately if he/she feels dizzy or experiences any pain

14. Place the tip of the nozzle into the EAM entrance and, using the foot control, direct a stream of water along the roof of the EAM and towards the posterior wall (directed towards the back of the patient's head). If you consider the entrance to the EAM as a clock face, you would direct the water at 11 o'clock in the right ear and 1 o'clock in the left ear. Increase the pressure control gradually if there is difficulty removing the wax. It is advisable that a maximum of two reservoirs of water is used in any one irrigation procedure

15. If the wax is not removed within five minutes of irrigation, it may be worthwhile moving on to the other ear (if irrigation required), as the introduction of water via the irrigating procedure will soften the wax and you can retry irrigation after about 15 minutes

16. Periodically inspect the EAM with the otoscope and inspect the solution running into the receiver

17. After removal of wax, dry excess water from the meatus

18. Examine the ear, both meatus and tympanic membrane, and treat as required following specific guidelines, or refer to a doctor if necessary

19. Decontaminate hands using correct hand hygiene techniques

20. Give advice regarding ear care and any relevant information

21. Document the procedure and findings

22. If any abnormality is found a referral should be made to the Doctor or ENT

Note: Irrigation should never cause pain. If the patient complains of pain - stop immediately. Follow manufacturer's guidelines and local policy for cleaning, disinfecting and calibrating the irrigator

37. Ear Swab Guidelines

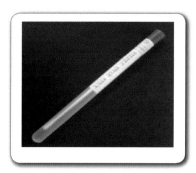

Equipment

- Non sterile gloves
- Apron
- Sterile swabs with transport medium
- Microbiology request forms

Procedure

1. Explain the procedure to the patient and gain informed consent

2. Ensure no antibiotics or other therapeutic drops have been used in the aural region 3 hours before taking the swab

3. Set up the equipment

4. Decontaminate hands using correct hand hygiene techniques

5. Position patient comfortably in a chair or on couch

6. Apply apron and gloves

7. Remove swab from outer packaging and place at the entrance to the auditory meatus and rotate gently

8. Remove cap from the transport tube

9. Carefully place swab into the transport tube, ensuring it is fully immersed in the transport medium. Ensure cap is secure. Label swab with full identifying details

10. Remove gloves and apron and wash/ decontaminate hands

11. Complete the microbiology request form with patient details, including relevant information such as exact site, nature of specimen and investigation required. Arrange prompt delivery to Lab or refrigerate at 4 – 8 degrees Celsius

12. Document the procedure in the patients records

38. Eye Irrigation Guidelines

Used mainly to flush secretions, chemicals, and foreign bodies from the eye, eye irrigation also provides a way to administer medications for corneal and conjunctival disorders. In an emergency, tap water may serve as eye irrigation fluid. The amount of solution needed to irrigate an eye depends on the contaminant. For minor eye irritations eye irrigation NACL solution pods (20mls) may be instilled by hand, however, secretions and foreign bodies require a moderate volume and major chemical burns require a copious amount. Usually, an IV bottle or bag of normal saline solution (with IV tubing attached) supplies enough solution for continuous irrigation of a chemical burn.

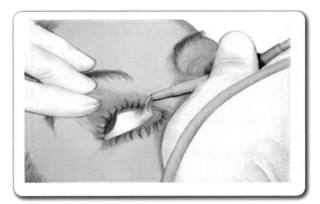

Equipment

- Sterile dressing pack

- Sterile water or normal saline solution for irrigation

- Tap water may be used in an emergency

- Universal pH indicator paper

- Receiver (Kidney dish)

- Towel

- Plastic cape

- IV fluid giving set and drip stand

- Warm water in a bowl to warm the irrigating fluid to tepid temperature

- Lint free Swabs

- Eye swabs (If required)

- Light source

- Disposable gloves (Sterile/non - sterile)

- Anaesthetic drops (if required)

Procedure

1. Explain the procedure and gain informed consent

2. Decontaminate hands using correct hand hygiene techniques and apply gloves.

3. If in situ - remove patient's contact lenses

4. In case of a chemical irritant: Ask the patient to look up. Draw lower lid down gently; insert pH indicator test paper at the junction of the middle and outer third of the lower lid. After strip is wet read against pH indicator score (after 30 seconds)

5. Instil anaesthetic drops if required

6. The patient should sit upright with head supported and tilted to the affected side

7. Drape the patients shoulders with a towel or if available a waterproof cape

8. Ask the patient to hold the receiver (kidney dish) against the cheek below the eye being irrigated

9. Prepare the irrigation fluid to the appropriate temperature by placing in the bowl of warm water until warmed

10. Hang the irrigation fluid on the drip stand, connect the fluid to the giving set and prime the line

11. If there is any discharge, take an eye swab (following correct procedure)

12. Hold the patients eyelids apart, using the first and second fingers, against the orbital ridge. Do not press on the eyeball

13. Warn the patient that the flow of solution is going to start and pour a little onto the cheek first

14. Direct the flow of the fluid from the nasal corner outwards. Keep the fluid flow constant by adjusting the giving set roller clamp

15. Ask the patient to look up, down and from side to side while irrigating

16. Evert upper and lower lids whilst irrigating

17. Keep the flow of irrigation fluid constant

18. A foreign body may be removed successfully in a couple of moments but a chemical irritant requires minimum 15 minutes irrigation and preferably 30 minutes

19. When the eye has been totally irrigated, ask the patient to close the eyes and use a lint free swab to dry the lids

20. In the case of a chemical burn/irritant check pH of patient's eye 5 minutes after completion of the irrigation. If outside normal range (7 - 7.5) repeat irrigation. If pH is within normal range check again after ½ hour to verify reading

21. Once the procedure is complete take the receiver from the patient and dry the cheek

22. Make the patient comfortable

23. Remove and dispose of equipment following correct protocol

24. Decontaminate hands using correct hand hygiene techniques

25. Document the intervention in the patient's notes

26. Discuss with the patient any changes post procedure; report any adverse effects/ findings to the doctor

27. In chemical: alkali and acid burns, refer the patient to an ophthalmologist for assessment

39. Eye Swab Guidelines

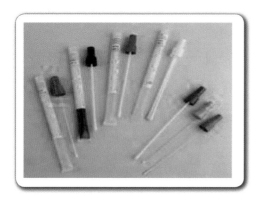

Equipment

- Non sterile gloves
- Apron
- Sterile swabs (bacterial or viral) with transport medium
- Microbiology request forms

Procedure

1. Explain the procedure to the patient and gain informed consent

2. Set up the equipment

3. Decontaminate hands using correct hand hygiene techniques

4. Position patient comfortably in a chair or on couch

5. Apply apron and gloves

6. Remove appropriate swab (s) (Bacterial/Viral) from outer packaging

7. Ask patient to look upwards

8. Hold the swab parallel to the cornea and gently rub the conjunctiva in the lower eyelids from the nasal side outwards

9. If swabbing for chlamydia, apply slightly more pressure when swabbing

10. If both eyes are to be swabbed, label swabs right and left accordingly

11. Remove cap from the transport tube

12. Carefully place swab into the transport tube, ensuring it is fully immersed in the transport medium. Ensure cap is secure. Label swab with full identifying details

13. Remove gloves and apron and wash/ decontaminate hands

14. Complete the microbiology request form with patient details, including relevant information such as exact site, nature of specimen and investigation required. Arrange delivery to the laboratory

15. Document the procedure in the patients notes

40. Throat Swab Guidelines

Equipment

- Non sterile gloves
- Apron
- Sterile swabs (bacterial or viral) with transport medium
- Tongue spatula/ depressor
- Light source
- Microbiology request forms

Procedure

1. Explain the procedure to the patient and gain informed consent
2. Set up the equipment
3. Decontaminate hands using correct hand hygiene techniques
4. Position patient comfortably in a chair or on couch
5. Apply apron and gloves
6. Remove appropriate swab (s) (Bacterial/Viral) from outer packaging
7. Ask patient to sit upright facing a strong light, tilt head backwards, open mouth and stick out tongue
8. Depress tongue with a spatula and ask patient to say 'Ah'
9. Quickly but gently roll the swab over any area of exudate or inflammation or over the tonsils and posterior pharynx
10. Carefully withdraw the swab, avoiding touching any other area of the mouth or tongue
11. Remove cap from the transport tube
12. Carefully place swab into the transport tube, ensuring it is fully immersed in the transport medium. Ensure cap is secure. Label swab with full identifying details
13. Remove gloves and apron and wash/ decontaminate hands
14. Complete the microbiology request form with patient details, including relevant information such as exact site, nature of specimen and investigation required. Arrange delivery to the laboratory
15. Document the procedure in the patients notes

41. Nasal Swab Guidelines

Equipment

- Non sterile gloves
- Apron
- Sterile bacterial or viral swabs with transport medium
- 0.9% NACL
- Microbiology request forms

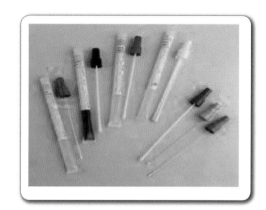

Procedure

1. Explain the procedure to the patient and gain informed consent
2. Set up the equipment
3. Decontaminate hands using correct hand hygiene techniques
4. Position patient comfortably in a chair or on the couch
5. Apply apron and gloves
6. Remove swab from outer packaging, ask patient to tilt head backwards
7. Moisten swab with sterile saline
8. Insert swab into the anterior nares with the tip directed upwards and gently rotate
9. Repeat the procedure with the same swab in the other nostril
10. Remove cap from the transport tube
11. Carefully place swab into the transport tube, ensuring it is fully immersed in the transport medium. Ensure cap is secure. Label swab with full identifying details
12. Provide the patient with a tissue
13. Remove gloves and apron and wash/ decontaminate hands
14. Complete the microbiology request form with patient details, including relevant information such as exact site, nature of specimen and investigation required.
15. If sample taken for screening: state clearly on the microbiology request form example MRSA screening
16. Arrange prompt delivery to the laboratory
17. Document the procedure in the patients records

42. Skin Swab Guidelines

Equipment

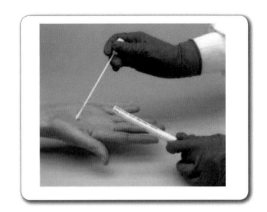

- Non sterile gloves
- Apron
- Sterile swabs (bacterial or viral) with transport medium
- Microbiology request forms
- Scalpel blade /U blade (trained practitioners only)

Procedure

1. Explain the procedure to the patient and gain informed consent

2. Set up the equipment

3. Decontaminate hands using correct hand hygiene techniques

4. Position patient comfortably

5. Apply apron and gloves

6. Remove appropriate swab (s) (Bacterial/Viral) from outer packaging

7. For cutaneous sampling (for screening/ example groin) moisten swab with sterile saline and roll one swab along the area of the skin along the inside of the thighs closest to the genitalia

8. For suspected fungal infection, skin scrapings should be obtained with a scalpel blade. Gently scrape, do not cause bleeding

9. For swab specimens, remove cap from the transport tube

10. Carefully place swab into the transport tube, ensuring it is fully immersed in the transport medium. Ensure cap is secure. Label swab with full identifying details

11. For skin scrapings, transfer scrapings into a sterile container

12. Remove gloves and apron and wash/ decontaminate hands Complete the microbiology request form with patient details, including relevant information such as exact site, nature of specimen and investigation required. Arrange delivery to the laboratory (Keep at room temperature)

13. Document the procedure in the patients notes

43. Penile Swab Guidelines

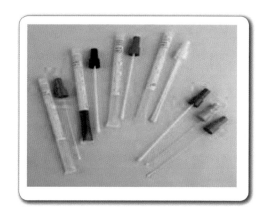

Equipment

- Non sterile gloves
- Apron
- Sterile swabs (bacterial or viral) with transport medium
- Microbiology request forms

Procedure

1. Explain the procedure to the patient and gain informed consent
2. The patient should not have passed urine for at least 1 hour
3. Set up the equipment
4. Decontaminate hands using correct hand hygiene techniques
5. Position patient comfortably on the couch bed
6. Apply apron and gloves
7. Remove appropriate swab (s) (Bacterial/Viral) from outer packaging
8. Retract prepuce
9. Press the swab gently through the urethral meatus and rotate gently
10. Remove cap from the transport tube
11. Carefully place swab into the transport tube, ensuring it is fully immersed in the transport medium. Ensure cap is secure. Label swab with full identifying details
12. Remove gloves and apron and wash/ decontaminate hands
13. Complete the microbiology request form with patient details, including relevant information such as exact site, nature of specimen and investigation required. Arrange delivery to the laboratory
14. Document the procedure in the patients notes

44. Rectal Swab Guidelines

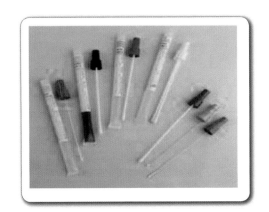

Equipment

- Non sterile gloves
- Apron
- Sterile swabs (bacterial or viral) with transport medium
- Microbiology request forms

Procedure

1. Explain the procedure to the patient and gain informed consent

2. Set up the equipment

3. Decontaminate hands using correct hand hygiene techniques

4. Position patient comfortably on the couch bed. Ensure privacy

5. Apply apron and gloves

6. Remove appropriate swab (s) (Bacterial/Viral) from outer packaging

7. Pass the swab with care, through the anus into the rectum and rotate gently

8. If specimen is for suspected threadworm, take swab from the perineal area

9. Remove cap from the transport tube

10. Carefully place swab into the transport tube, ensuring it is fully immersed in the transport medium. Ensure cap is secure. Label swab with full identifying details

11. Remove gloves and apron and decontaminate hands using correct hand hygiene techniques

12. Complete the microbiology request form with patient details, including relevant information such as exact site, nature of specimen and investigation required. Arrange delivery to the laboratory

13. Document the procedure in the patients notes

45. Adult Peripheral Venepuncture Guidelines

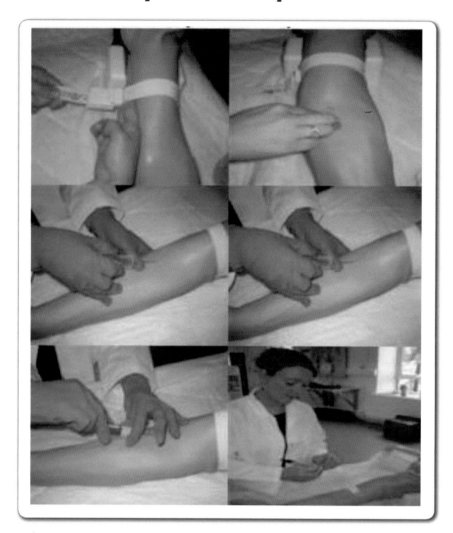

Equipment

- Clinical tray with disposal sharps unit
- Non - sterile powder free disposable gloves
- Disposable tourniquet (single use)
- Large 70% isopropyl alcohol swabs
- Gauze swabs
- Sterile disposable double - ended vacutainer needle/ Plastic vacutainer holder or vacuette winged blood collecting device
- Appropriate blood specimen tubes
- Sterile adhesive plaster / hypoallergenic tape
- Laboratory specimen requisition forms
- Plastic specimen laboratory bag or biohazard bag (where applicable)

Procedure

1. Explain the procedure to the patient and gain consent

2. Decontaminate hands using correct hand hygiene techniques

3. Apply the tourniquet. The tourniquet should be tight enough to impede venous return while not affecting arterial flow. Allow time for the veins to fill. Ensure that the tourniquet is not applied for longer than clinically indicated

4. Make a full assessment of the patient's veins. Inspect the area for phlebitis, infection or oedema, bruised or inflamed veins, or any veins that have undergone multiple punctures. These veins are to be avoided

5. Palpate the veins most likely to be used. Stroking the vein and observing the venous refills are helpful in determining the condition of the vein

6. Assess and select the most appropriate vein.

7. Select the device based on vein size and location

8. Decontaminate hands using correct hand hygiene techniques

9. Put on well - fitting powder free disposable gloves

10. Clean the insertion site using a 70% isopropyl alcohol impregnated swab for a minimum of 30 seconds and allow to air dry for a minimum of 30 seconds. Do not re - palpate or touch the skin

11. Remove the needle from the packaging and inspect it for any faults

12. Stabilize the vein by applying manual traction on the skin a few centimetres below the proposed insertion site using the non - dominant hand

13. Ensure the needle tip is in the bevel up position. Place the device directly over or to the side of the vein and insert the needle smoothly through the skin at a 30 degree angle according to the depth of the vein

14. As soon as puncture of the vein wall is felt, level off the needle by decreasing the angle of the needle to the skin. If using a winged blood collection device, a flashback of blood is seen in the tubing

15. Slightly advance the needle in order to stabilize it within the vein if possible

16. Gently release the skin tension. If using a winged device, tape one wing to stabilize the device if necessary

17. Do not exert any pressure on the needle

18. Keeping the needle and vacutainer holder steady in position, attach the appropriate blood specimen tube onto the needle inside the holder and withdraw the blood

19. Samples may be obtained one after another by removing the filled tube and replacing it with another. Ensure that the tube is correctly filled to the fill mark on the tube label

20. Collect samples in the following order as recommended by manufacturer's guidelines
    - Non - additive tubes
    - Coagulation
    - Serum
    - Heparin
    - EDTA
    - Glucose
    - All others

21. During filling of the last tube, release and remove the tourniquet to decrease the pressure within the vein

22. It may be necessary to release the tourniquet at the beginning of the sampling as inaccurate measurements may be caused by haemostasis. This is specific when drawing blood to assess calcium levels

23. Remove the last specimen tube from the holder, prior to removing the needle

24. Place a gauze swab over the puncture point. Remove the needle but do not apply pressure until the needle has been fully removed

25. Apply firm digital pressure directly over the puncture site until bleeding has stopped

26. The patient may apply pressure with the fingers but should be discouraged from bending the arm if a vein in the antecubital fossa is used

27. After a sample has been taken, it is important that the sample be gently inverted 4 - 6 times. This will allow the sample to mix with the additive and reduce the risk of clots forming in the tube, which can later break during centrifugation and cause haemolysis

28. All specimen tubes must be labelled immediately with the relevant patient details

29. Inspect the puncture site before applying a dressing

30. Apply an adhesive plaster/ dressing

31. Ensure the patient is comfortable and pain free

32. Discard waste, making sure it is disposed of in the correct sharps containers and appropriate waste bags

33. Remove gloves and dispose of appropriately, clean hands according to correct hand hygiene technique

34. If a sample tube contains an additive, invert the tube to mix the blood and the additive to prevent clotting or aid accurate measurement

35. Place specimens in sealable section of the plastic laboratory transport bag. Place completed blood request forms/ in appropriate pocket of laboratory transport bag

36. Follow local procedures for collection and transport of specimens to the laboratory

References
Health Service Executive (2010). National Clinical Policy and Procedural Guidelines for Nurses and Midwives undertaking Peripheral Cannulation in Adults. HSE: Dublin

Note: Do not exceed two attempts. If unsuccessful after two attempts another suitably trained practitioner should perform the venepuncture

46. Blood Vacutainers and Specimen Containers

Vacutainer Blood Bottles

- **Cap Colour:** Yellow Clotted **Anticoagulant:** (No Anticoagulant) **Test:** All serum tests
- **Cap Colour:** Grey **Anticoagulant:** Fluoride Oxalate **Test:** Blood Glucose
- **Cap Colour:** Purple **Anticoagulant:** E.D.T.A **Test:** FBC/ESR
- **Cap Colour:** Green **Anticoagulant:** Lithium Heparin **Test:** Plasma tests
- **Cap Colour:** Blue **Anticoagulant:** Sodium Citrate **Test:** Coagulation tests
- **Cap Colour:** Pink **Anticoagulant:** E.D.T.A **Test:** X Match

Other Containers

- **Containers:** Boric Acid Container (Red Top) **Tests/Specimens:** Urine (Microscopy Culture) Urinary Antigen (Legionnella/Pneumococcal)
- **Containers:** Sterile Universal (polypropylene) 30ml **Tests/Specimens:** CSF, Aspirates, Sterile fluids, Catheter tips, Pus samples, Sputa, BAL
- **Containers:** 250 ml Sterile Universal (polypropylene) **Tests/Specimens:** Early Morning Urine(TB)
- **Containers:** Sterile Universal (with Spoon) **Tests/Specimens:** Faeces/ Stool
- **Containers:** Amplicor Swab (Chlamydia) **Tests/Specimens:** Chlamydia PCR
- **Containers:** Amies Transport Swab (Blue top) **Tests/Specimens:** All Wounds, Genital specimens MRSA/VRE screens. Upper respiratory Tract specimens.
- **Containers:** High Nasal/Pernasal (Blue top wire shaft)**Tests/Specimens:** Pertussis
- **Containers:** ENT Swab (orange top charcoal) **Tests/Specimens:** Inner Ear/Sinus Swab
- **Containers:** Viral Transport Medium (Pink top) **Tests/Specimens:** Viral Culture

Blood Culture Bottle Sets

- **Colour:** Blue and Purple **Blood Culture:** Aerobic/Anaerobic
- **Colour:** Green and purple **Blood Culture:** Fan Aerobic/Anaerobic
- **Colour:** Yellow **Blood Culture:** Paediatric

Source: Health Service Executive (2018). Acute Hospital Laboratory Supplies. Type of Specimen Containers. HSE: Dublin.

47. Intravenous Cannulation Guidelines

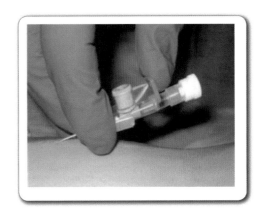

Equipment

- Intravenous tray with sharps disposal unit
- Powder free, non - sterile gloves
- Disposable tourniquet
- Various gauge sizes of cannula Large 70% isopropyl alcohol swabs
- A semi - permeable transparent adhesive dressing
- Clave connector/ intravenous bung
- Primed extension tubing or intravenous infusion set and solution (if necessary)
- 5mls of 0.9% Sodium Chloride solution
- Sterile 10ml syringe

Procedure

1. Explain the procedure to the patient and gain consent.
2. Decontaminate hands using correct hand hygiene techniques
3. Expose site. Do not shave skin over the site: excessive hair may be clipped if necessary
4. Ensure a comfortable position for practitioner and patient, making sure there is adequate lighting and ventilation
5. Apply the tourniquet. Ensure that the tourniquet is not applied for any longer than clinically indicated.
6. Identify the vein - assess, palpate and select
7. Select the cannula device based on the vein size and location
8. Decontaminate hands using correct hand hygiene techniques
9. Put on powder free, well - fitting non - sterile disposable gloves

10. Clean the insertion site using a 70% isopropyl alcohol impregnated swab for a minimum of 30 seconds and allow to air dry for a minimum of 30 seconds. Do not re - palpate or touch the skin

11. Remove the cannula device from the packaging and inspect for any faults

12. Anchor the vein by applying manual traction on the skin a few centimetres below the proposed site of insertion, using the non - dominant hand

13. Ensure the cannula is in the bevel up position. Place the device directly over the vein and insert the cannula smoothly through the skin at a 30 degree angle according to the depth of the vein

14. Wait for the first flashback of blood into the flashback chamber of the stylet. This confirms entry of the needle tip into the vein

15. Level the device by decreasing the angle between the cannula and the skin and advance the cannula slightly to ensure entry to the lumen of the vein

16. Withdraw the stylet gradually and observe for blood in the cannula tubing

17. Maintain skin traction with the non - dominant hand slowly advance the cannula off the stylet and into the vein with the dominant hand

18. Release tourniquet and apply digital pressure to the vein above the cannula tip and remove the stylet

19. Immediately dispose of the stylet into an appropriate sharps container

20. Attach a clave connector/ injection cap / pre - flushed extension set /or administration set to the cannula hub using aseptic techniques

21. Secure wings of the cannula with strips of sterile narrow adhesive tape

22. Place a sterile semi - permeable transparent dressing over the catheter site ensuring the cannula is secure. Ensure the entry site of the cannula is clearly visible. Initial and document the dressing with date of insertion

23. Blood samples required for analysis must be drawn before flushing the cannula with saline. It is recommended that the initial sample be discarded prior to securing further samples. After any flushing or medication has been administered, the cannula may no longer be used for blood collection

24. Flush the cannula with 5mls of normal saline 0.9%, to check patency, clear the cannula and minimise the risk of infection

25. Observe the site for signs of swelling or leakage and ask the patient if any discomfort or pain is felt

26. Discard waste, making sure it is disposed of in the correct sharps containers and appropriate waste bags

27. Remove gloves and dispose of appropriately

28. Decontaminate hands using correct hand hygiene technique

29. Ensure the patient is comfortable

30. Document procedure in the relevant nursing / appropriate notes.

31. Do not exceed two attempts. If unsuccessful after two attempts, it is recommended that another suitably trained practitioner perform the intravenous cannulation.

References
Health Service Executive (2010). A Guiding Framework for Education, Training and Competence Validation in Venepuncture and Peripheral Intravenous Cannulation for Nurses and Midwives. HSE: Dublin.

48. Peripheral Intravenous Cannula Removal

Equipment

- A clean clinical tray
- Small kidney dish for Healthcare Risk Waste (placed in tray) or use clinical tray with 2 integrated compartments (one to be used for waste)
- Disposable non sterile sheet (optional in case of blood spillage)
- Personal Protective Equipment (PPE) e.g. 2 pairs of well - fitting non - sterile gloves, protective plastic apron, safety goggles/visor/mask with eye shield
- Adhesive remover/spray/cleanser
- Sterile gauze
- Sterile waterproof plaster or dressing

Procedure

1. Confirm indication for removal of peripheral intravenous cannula
2. Disinfect a clean clinical tray using 70% alcohol (or equivalent as per local guidelines)
3. Collect the appropriate equipment and inspect it's integrity
4. Decontaminate hands using correct hand hygiene techniques
5. Check patient's identification
6. Explain the procedure, check for allergies to dressings and obtain informed consent to remove the cannula
7. Open the sterile gauze and sterile dressing using the packaging as a sterile field
8. Ensure the patient is in a comfortable position
9. Examine the peripheral intravenous cannulation site and surrounding area for signs of infection or infiltration
10. Stop intravenous infusion if in place
11. Apply gloves (apron and eye protection if required)
12. Remove the outer dressing, using adhesive remover if necessary and place in kidney dish or compartment in clinical tray for waste
13. Remove the taping from around the cannula and place in kidney dish or compartment in clinical tray for waste

Cannula Removal

14. Slowly remove the cannula. With sterile gauze, apply gentle pressure as the cannula tip is removed

15. Inspect the cannula length and integrity on removal

16. Place cannula into kidney dish or compartment in clinical tray for waste

17. Maintain gentle pressure to peripheral intravenous site and hold in place for two to three minutes

18. Inspect Peripheral intravenous cannulation site for evidence of infection or inflammation

19. Apply sterile gauze dressing or sterile plaster

20. Remove gloves and eye protection if applicable and place in the clinical tray

21. Decontaminate hands using correct hand hygiene techniques

After Care

22. Inform the patient of possible complications and advise to report same

23. Ensure the patient is in a comfortable position and reassure

24. Document the procedure, communicate and inform relevant staff

25. Apply gloves and bring tray with used items to the dirty utility

26. Dispose of healthcare risk and non - risk waste appropriately

27. Clean and disinfect the clinical tray and kidney dish if reusable

28. Clean and disinfect reusable eye shield as per manufacturer's instructions if applicable

29. Remove gloves and apron if applicable and carry out appropriate hand hygiene technique

30. Organise for reinsertion of a peripheral intravenous cannula if required

References
Health Service Executive (2010). A Guiding Framework for Education, Training and Competence Validation in Venepuncture and Peripheral Intravenous Cannulation for Nurses and Midwives. HSE: Dublin

49. Medications

1. Oral Administration Guidelines

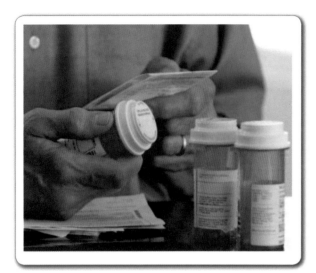

Equipment

- Medication to be administered
- Medication record sheet
- Prescription chart
- Glass of water
- Disposable medication container
- PPE example gloves if required for specific medication example cytotoxic medication

Procedure

1. Explain the procedure and gain informed consent
2. Decontaminate hands using correct hand hygiene techniques
3. Before administering any prescribed medication, check that it is due and has not already been given
4. Carry out any required assessment such as pulse, BP, respiration, temperature
5. Check that the prescription is complete, correct and legible
6. Before administering any prescribed medication look at the prescription chart and check the following
   - Correct patient
   - Correct medication
   - Correct dose
   - Date and time of administration
   - Diluent as appropriate
   - Validity of prescription
   - Signature of prescriber
   - Prescription is legible

If any of these pieces of information are missing, unclear or illegible then the nurse should not proceed with administration and should consult with the prescriber

7. Select the required medication and check the expiry date

8. Empty the required dose into a medicine container. Avoid touching the preparation

9. Check the patients identity by confirming their name and date of birth or by checking their name band if necessary

10. Check the patients allergy status

11. Evaluate the patients knowledge about the medication and explain the use, action, dose and potential side effects of the medication

12. Administer the medication as prescribed.

13. Offer a glass of water and assist the patient where necessary

14. Stay with the patient until they have swallowed all of the medication

15. Record/ document the medication given and sign the prescription record

16. Wash/ decontaminate hands according to correct hand hygiene techniques

References
Health Service Executive (2012). Guidelines for the administration of medications. HSE: Dublin.

2. Administering Intramuscular Injection Guidelines

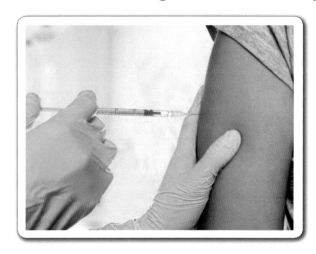

Equipment

- Needle (correct gauge)
- Syringe containing prepared IM medication
- Clean receiver or tray
- Alcohol swab
- Non - sterile gloves
- Apron Prescription chart
- Sharps bin

Procedure

1. Explain the procedure and gain informed consent
2. Decontaminate hands using correct hand hygiene techniques
3. Before administering any prescribed medication, check that it is due and has not already been given
4. Carry out any required assessment such as pulse, BP, respiration, temperature
5. Check that the prescription is complete, correct and legible
6. Before administering any prescribed medication look at the prescription chart and check the following
   - Correct patient
   - Correct medication
   - Correct dose
   - Date and time of administration
   - Diluent as appropriate
   - Validity of prescription
   - Signature of prescriber
   - Prescription is legible

If any of these pieces of information are missing, unclear or illegible then the nurse should not proceed with administration and should consult with the prescriber

7. Clean hands according to hand hygiene techniques. Apply apron and gloves.

8. Select and prepare the required medication and check the expiry date

9. Check the patients identity by confirming their name and date of birth or by checking their name band if necessary

10. Check the patients allergy status

11. Evaluate the patients knowledge about the medication and explain the use, action, dose and potential side effects of the medication

12. Ensure privacy. Ask the patient to remove the appropriate garment to expose the injection site and assist patient into the correct position

13. Assess the injection site for signs of inflammation, oedema, infection and skin lesions

14. Choose the appropriate injection site. Clean the injection site with a 70% isopropyl alcohol swab for 30 seconds and allow to dry for 30 seconds

15. With the non - dominant hand, stretch the skin slightly around the injection site

16. Holding the syringe in the dominant hand like a dart, inform the patient and quickly plunge the needle at an angle of 90 degrees into the skin until about 1 cm of the needle is left showing

17. Pull back the plunger. If no blood is aspirated depress the plunger at approximately 1ml every 10 seconds and inject the drug slowly. If blood appears withdraw the needle completely, replace it and begin again. Explain to the patient what has occurred

18. Wait 10 seconds before withdrawing the needle

19. Withdraw the needle quickly. Apply gentle pressure but do not massage the site

20. Apply a small plaster if required over the puncture site

21. Where appropriate activate safety device. Ensure that all sharps are disposed of correctly in the sharps bin and other equipment in the correct waste

22. Record/ document the medication given and sign the prescription record

23. Wash/ decontaminate hands according to correct hand hygiene techniques

References
Health Service Executive (2012). Guidelines for the administration of medications. HSE: Dublin.

3. Administering Subcutaneous Injection Guidelines

Equipment

- Patient's prescription
- Syringe containing the prepared medication
  Alcohol /skin cleansing swab
- Gloves and apron
- Cotton swab/ gauze
- Sharps bin

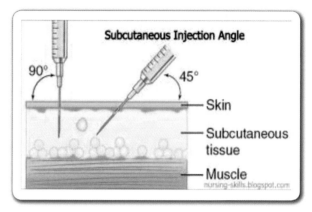

Procedure

1. Explain the procedure and gain informed consent

2. Decontaminate hands using correct hand hygiene techniques

3. Before administering any prescribed medication, check that it is due and has not already been given. Check the patients allergy status

4. Carry out any required assessments such as pulse, BP, respiration, temperature

5. Check that the prescription is complete, correct and legible

6. Before administering any prescribed medication look at the prescription chart and check the following

   - Correct patient
   - Correct medication
   - Correct dose
   - Date and time of administration
   - Diluent as appropriate
   - Validity of prescription
   - Signature of prescriber
   - Prescription is legible

If any of these pieces of information are missing, unclear or illegible then the nurse should not proceed with administration and should consult with the prescriber

7. Assist the patient into the required position. Ensure privacy.

8. Remove appropriate garment to expose injection site

9. Assess the injection site for signs of inflammation, oedema, infection and skin lesions

10. Decontaminate hands and apply non sterile gloves and apron

11. Check unit volume of the injection. Ensure dose administered is consistent with prescription

12. Where appropriate, clean the injection site with a 70% isopropyl alcohol swab

13. Remove the cover from the needle taking care not to contaminate the needle

14. Gently pinch the skin up into a fold

15. Hold the syringe between the thumb and forefinger of the dominant hand as if grasping a dart

16. Introduce the needle quickly, but in a controlled manner all the way into the skin at a 45 degree angle (unless administering insulin when an angle of 90 degrees should be used) and release the grasped skin. The angle is important to allow all the medication to be injected into the fatty tissue. However in individuals with very little subcutaneous fat, the angle of injecting may vary

17. Inject the medication at a slow steady rate over 10 seconds by pushing the plunger to deliver the medication

18. Remove the needle rapidly

19. Using a cotton swab or gauze, briefly apply light pressure at the injection site. This will help lessen oozing or bleeding but do not rub or apply pressure to the area (Bruising)

    - Do not put the cap back on the needle
    - Discard the entire syringe in the sharps container supplied

20. Remove gloves and decontaminate hands using correct hand hygiene techniques

21. Document the procedure and dosage administered in the patients notes

4. Administering Subcutaneous, Anticoagulant Injections Guidelines

Subcutaneous anticoagulant injections (example innohep) are administered into the fatty layer of tissue just under the skin. The most common body areas used to give these injections are:

- Fleshy part of the thigh.
- Abdomen.

Contraindications

Do not use subcutaneous anticoagulants in the following instances;

- Allergy to its ingredients (benzyl alcohol, sodium metabisulphite) or to heparin
- History of decreased platelet count
- Bacterial infection of the heart
- Bleed easily or have conditions or diseases with a high risk of bleeding
- Blood clotting disorder which increases the risk of bleeding
- Cerebrovascular accident (e.g. stroke)
- Stomach or intestinal ulcer or an ulcerating cancer
- Uncontrolled, severe high blood pressure
- Eye disorders due to diabetes or bleeding
- Injury or surgery on the brain, spinal cord, eyes or ears
- Artificial heart valve
- A spinal/epidural anaesthesia and high doses of innohep increases the risk of bleeding

Interactions

Subcutaneous anticoagulants should be used with caution in patients taking oral anticoagulants, NSAIDS, platelet inhibitors and thrombolytic agents

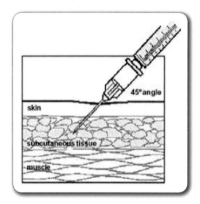

Equipment

- Patient's prescription chart
- Anticoagulant injection (check unit volume and ensure dose administered is consistent with prescription)
- Appropriate skin cleansing agent
- Gloves
- Cotton swab Sharps bin

Procedure

1. Explain the procedure and gain informed consent
2. Decontaminate hands using correct hand hygiene techniques
3. Before administering any prescribed medication, check that it is due and has not already been given. Check the patients allergy status
4. Carry out any required assessment such as pulse, BP, respiration, temperature
5. Check that the prescription is complete, correct and legible
6. Before administering any prescribed medication look at the prescription chart and check the following

   - Correct patient
   - Correct medication
   - Correct dose
   - Date and time of administration
   - Diluent as appropriate
   - Validity of prescription
   - Signature of prescriber
   - Prescription is legible

If any of these pieces of information are missing, unclear or illegible then the nurse should not proceed with administration and should consult with the prescriber

1. Take one of the pre - filled injections from the box. Ensure that the fluid inside the syringe is clear and free from particles
2. Check unit volume of the injection. Ensure dose administered is consistent with prescription and check that the medication is in date
3. Remove the cover from the needle taking care not to contaminate the needle. When injecting anticoagulant a small air bubble will be seen in the syringe. This can be left in the syringe for injecting.
4. Clean the area of skin using appropriate cleansing agent
5. Hold the syringe in one hand like a pencil or dart
6. Pinch the area of skin to be injected between the thumb and index finger.

7. Introduce the needle quickly, but in a controlled manner all the way into the skin at a 45 degree angle. The angle is important to allow all the medication to be injected into the fatty tissue. However in individuals with very little subcutaneous fat, the angle of injecting may vary

8. Let go of the pinched skin and inject the medication at a slow steady rate by pushing the plunger to deliver the medication.

9. Remove the needle slowly.

10. Using a cotton swab or gauze, briefly apply light pressure at the injection site. This will help lessen oozing or bleeding but do not rub or apply pressure to the area (Bruising)

11. Slight bruising at the injection site is common.

12. Disposal of the syringe

    - Do not put the cap back on the needle
    - Discard the entire syringe in the sharps container supplied

13. Remove gloves and wash/ decontaminate hands using correct hand hygiene techniques

14. Document the procedure and dosage administered in the patients notes

References
Royal Collage of Nursing (2017). Guidelines for the administration of subcutaneous anticoagulant medications. RCN: London.

5. Intradermal Injection, Administration Guidelines

Equipment

- Needle 25 – 27 G

- 1ml syringe containing medication

- Alcohol swab

- Non - sterile gloves

- Apron

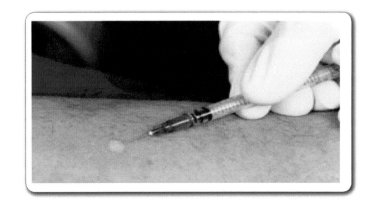

Procedure

1. Explain the procedure and gain informed consent

2. Decontaminate hands using correct hand hygiene techniques

3. Before administering any prescribed medication, check that it is due and has not already been given. Check the patients allergy status

4. Carry out any required assessments such as pulse, BP, respiration, temperature

5. Check that the prescription is complete, correct and legible

6. Before administering any prescribed medication look at the prescription chart and check the following

   - Correct patient

   - Correct medication

   - Correct dose

   - Date and time of administration

   - Diluent as appropriate

   - Validity of prescription

   - Signature of prescriber

   - Prescription is legible

If any of these pieces of information are missing, unclear or illegible then the nurse should not proceed with administration and should consult with the prescriber

7. Assist the patient into the required position. Ensure privacy

8. Remove appropriate garment to expose injection site

9. Assess the injection site for signs of inflammation, oedema, infection and skin lesions

10. Decontaminate hands and apply non sterile gloves and apron

11. Check unit volume of the injection. Ensure dose administered is consistent with prescription

12. Where appropriate, clean the injection site with a 70% isopropyl alcohol swab

13. Remove the needle sheath and hold syringe with the dominant hand with the bevel of the needle pointing up

14. With the non - dominant hand, stretch skin over the site with forefinger and thumb

15. With the needle almost against the patients skin, insert the needle into the skin at an angle of 10 – 15 degrees and advance through the epidermis so the needle tip can be seen through the skin

16. Inject medication slowly. It is not necessary to aspirate as the dermis is relatively avascular

17. While injecting medication, a bleb will form

18. Withdraw the needle rapidly

19. Using a cotton swab or gauze, briefly apply light pressure at the injection site, but do not rub or massage the area

20. Do not put the cap back on the needle. Where appropriate, activate safety device

21. Ensure that all sharps and non - sharp waste are disposed of safely and according to correct procedure

22. Remove gloves and decontaminate hands using correct hand hygiene techniques

23. Document the procedure and dosage administered in the patients notes

References
Health Service Executive (2012). Guidelines for the administration of medications. HSE: Dublin.

6. Medication Administration by Inhalation using a Metered Dose Inhaler Guidelines

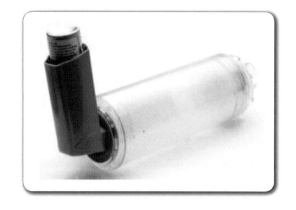

Equipment

- Metered Dose Inhaler Device (MDI) Spacer device

- Prescription chart

- Peak flow if required

Procedure

1. Explain the procedure and gain informed consent. Correct use of inhalers is essential and will be achieved only if this is carefully explained and demonstrated to the patient

2. Decontaminate hands using correct hand hygiene techniques

3. Before administering any prescribed medication, check that it is due and has not already been given

4. Carry out any required assessment such as pulse, BP, respiration, peak flow

5. Check that the prescription is complete, correct and legible

6. Before administering any prescribed medication look at the prescription chart and check the following

    - Correct patient
    - Correct medication
    - Correct dose
    - Date and time of administration
    - Diluent as appropriate
    - Validity of prescription
    - Signature of prescriber
    - Prescription is legible

If any of these pieces of information are missing, unclear or illegible then the nurse should not proceed with administration and should consult with the prescriber

7. Select the required inhaler, check the expiry date and that the device is clean and intact

8. Check the patients identity by confirming their name and date of birth or by checking their name band if necessary

9. Check the patients allergy status

10. Evaluate the patients knowledge about the medication and explain the use, action, dose and potential side effects of the medication

11. Administer the medication as prescribed.

12. Remove the mouthpiece cover from the inhaler

13. Shake inhaler well for 2 – 3 seconds

14. Sit the patient in an upright position

15. Without a spacer device: Ask the patient to take a deep breath and exhale completely. Open lips and place inhaler mouthpiece in mouth, closing lips tightly around it

16. With a spacer device: Insert MDI into end of the spacer device. Ask the patient to exhale and then grasp spacer mouthpiece with teeth and lips while holding inhaler

17. Ask patient to tip head back slightly, inhale slowly and deeply through the mouth while depressing canister fully

18. Instruct the patient to breathe in slowly for 2 - 3 seconds and hold their breath for approximately 10 seconds, then remove MDI from the mouth (if not using spacer) before exhaling slowly through pursed lips

19. Instruct the patient to wait 20 - 30 seconds between inhalations of same medications or 2– 5 minutes between inhalation of different medications

20. If steroid medication is administered, ask the patient to rinse their mouth with water approximately 2 minutes after inhaling the dose

21. Clean any equipment used and discard all used disposable equipment in appropriate waste

22. Record/ document the medication given and sign the prescription record

23. Wash/decontaminate hands according to correct hand hygiene techniques

Source: Health Service Executive (2012). Guidelines for the administration of medications. HSE: Dublin.

7. Administration by Inhalation using a Nebuliser Guidelines

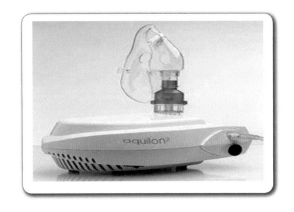

Equipment

- Nebuliser medication
- Nebuliser machine and disposable tubing
- Disposable/ individual facemask or mouthpiece
- Prescription chart
- Peak flow (If required)

Procedure

1. Explain the procedure and gain informed consent. Correct use of nebulisers is essential and will be achieved only if this is carefully explained and demonstrated to the patient

2. Decontaminate hands using correct hand hygiene techniques

3. Before administering any prescribed medication, check that it is due and has not already been given

4. Carry out any required assessment such as pulse, BP, respiration, peak flow

5. Check that the prescription is complete, correct and legible

6. Before administering any prescribed medication look at the prescription chart and check the following

    - Correct patient
    - Correct medication
    - Correct dose
    - Date and time of administration
    - Diluent as appropriate
    - Validity of prescription
    - Signature of prescriber
    - Prescription is legible

If any of these pieces of information are missing, unclear or illegible then the nurse should not proceed with administration and should consult with the prescriber

7. Select the prescribed nebuliser medication, check the expiry date and that the nebuliser machine is clean, intact and in good working order

8. Check the patients identity by confirming their name and date of birth or by checking their name band if necessary

9. Check the patients allergy status

10. Evaluate the patients knowledge about the medication and explain the use, action, dose and potential side effects of the medication

11. Administer the medication as prescribed and only one medication at a time

12. Sit the patient in an upright position

13. Assemble the nebuliser equipment as per manufacturer's instructions

14. Add the prescribed medication and diluent if required to the nebuliser

15. Attach the mouthpiece or facemask to the nebuliser machine

16. If the patient has a clinical need pulse oximetry should be carried out for the duration of the procedure

17. If the patient is hypercapnic or acidotic (example COPD), the nebuliser should be driven by medical air, not oxygen

18. Ask the patient to hold the mouthpiece between the lips or apply the facemask and take a slow deep breath. After inspiration the patient should pause briefly and exhale

19. Turn on the nebuliser machine, and observe that sufficient mist is formed

20. The patient should continue to breathe as instructed during the procedure until the nebulised medication is complete

21. Optimal nebulisation takes approximately 10 minutes

22. Check peak flow post nebuliser if required

23. Once completed, clean the equipment and dispose of any disposable equipment/ tubing in the appropriate waste

24. Record/ document the medication given and sign the prescription record

25. Wash/decontaminate hands according to correct hand hygiene techniques

Source: Health Service Executive (2012). Guidelines for the administration of medications. HSE: Dublin

8. Transdermal Application Guidelines

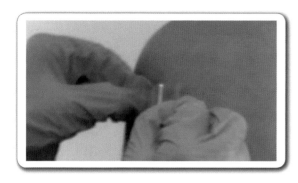

Equipment

- Transdermal patch
- Medication record sheet
- Prescription chart
- Non-sterile gloves
- Apron

Procedure

1. Explain the procedure and gain informed consent
2. Decontaminate hands using correct hand hygiene techniques
3. Before administering any prescribed medication, check that it is due and has not already been given
4. Carry out any required assessment such as pulse, BP, temperature, respiration
5. Check that the prescription is complete, correct and legible
6. Before administering any prescribed medication check the following

    - Correct patient
    - Correct medication
    - Correct dose
    - Date and time of administration
    - Diluent as appropriate
    - Validity of prescription
    - Signature of prescriber
    - Prescription is legible

If any of these pieces of information are missing, unclear or illegible then the nurse should not proceed with administration and should consult with the prescriber

7. Select the required medication- Transdermal patch and check the expiry date
8. Check the patients identity by confirming their name and date of birth or by checking their name band if necessary

9. Check the patients allergy status

10. Evaluate the patients knowledge about the medication and explain the use, action, dose and potential side effects of the medication

11. Assist the patient into the correct position and ensure privacy

12. Expose the area of skin that requires the transdermal patch and if necessary cover the patient with a towel or disposable sheet

13. Apply gloves and assess the condition of the skin. Do not apply to skin that is oily, burnt, cut or irritated

14. Where necessary, remove the used patch and fold it in half, adhesive sides inwards, place in the clinical waste

15. Carefully remove the new patch from its protective cover and hold it by the edge without touching the adhesive edges

16. Apply the patch immediately to the correct area of skin (following product guidelines) pressing firmly with the palm of the hand for up to 10 seconds, making sure the patch sticks well around the edges

17. Date and initial the patch

18. Remove gloves and apron and dispose of waste appropriately

19. Wash/ decontaminate hands according to correct hand hygiene techniques

20. Document the medication given and sign the prescription record

Source: Health Service Executive (2012). Guidelines for the administration of medications. HSE: Dublin

9. Eye Medication Administration Guidelines

Equipment

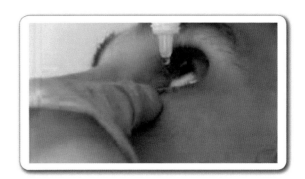

- Eye drops to be administered
- Non-sterile powder free gloves
- Low linting swabs
- Sterile 0.9% NACL or water
- Eye swab
- Prescription chart

Procedure

1. Explain the procedure and gain informed consent
2. Decontaminate hands using correct hand hygiene techniques
3. Before administering any prescribed medication, check that it is due and has not already been given
4. Carry out any required assessment such as pulse, BP, temperature, respiration
5. Check that the prescription is complete, correct and legible
6. Before administering any prescribed medication look at the prescription chart and check the following
    - Correct patient
    - Correct medication
    - Correct dose
    - Date and time of administration
    - Diluent as appropriate
    - Validity of prescription
    - Signature of prescriber
    - Prescription is legible

If any of these pieces of information are missing, unclear or illegible then the nurse should not proceed with administration and should consult with the prescriber

7. Select the required eye drop/ ointment medication and check the expiry date

8. Check the patients identity by confirming their name and date of birth or by checking their name band if necessary

9. Check the patients allergy status

10. Evaluate the patients knowledge about the medication and explain the use, action, dose and potential side effects of the medication

11. Ask the patient to sit back with neck slightly hyperextended or to lie down

12. Wash hands according to hand hygiene techniques and apply gloves and gown

13. If there is any discharge proceed as for eye swabbing (see separate guidelines). If any crusting or drainage is present around the eye, gently wash away with sterile water or 0.9% NACL on a swab. Always wipe from the inner to the outer canthus

14. Administer the medication as prescribed

15. Ask the patient to look at the ceiling and carefully pull the skin below the affected eye using a wet swab to expose the conjunctival sac

16. If administering both drops and ointment, administer drops first

17. Either: Administer the prescribed number of drops, holding an eye dropper 1-2 cm above the eye. If the patient blinks or closes their eye repeat the procedure. Or: Apply a thin strip of ointment along the inner edge of the lower eyelid or conjunctiva from the nasal corner outwards. If there is excess medication on the eyelid, wipe it from the inner to outer canthus

18. Ask the patient to close their eyes and keep them closed for 1-2 minutes

19. Explain to the patient that they may have blurred vision for a few minutes after application

20. Clean the equipment used according to manufacturer's recommendations and discard all disposable equipment, gloves and apron in the appropriate/ clinical waste

21. Document the medication given and sign the prescription record

22. Decontaminate hands according to correct hand hygiene techniques

Source: Health Service Executive (2012). Guidelines for the administration of medications. HSE: Dublin.

10. Ear Drop Administration Guidelines

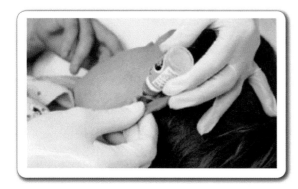

Equipment

- Ear drops to be administered
- Non-sterile gloves
- Apron
- Tissues
- Cotton tipped applicator
- Prescription chart

Procedure

1. Explain the procedure and gain informed consent
2. Decontaminate hands using correct hand hygiene techniques
3. Before administering any prescribed medication, check that it is due and has not already been given
4. Carry out any required assessments such as pulse, BP, temperature, respiration
5. Check that the prescription is complete, correct and legible
6. Before administering any prescribed medication look at the prescription chart and check the following

   - Correct patient
   - Correct medication
   - Correct dose
   - Date and time of administration
   - Diluent as appropriate
   - Validity of prescription
   - Signature of prescriber
   - Prescription is legible

   If any of these pieces of information are missing, unclear or illegible then the nurse should not proceed with administration and should consult with the prescriber

7. Select the required ear drop medication and check the expiry date

8. Check the patients identity by confirming their name and date of birth or by checking their name band if necessary

9. Check the patients allergy status

10. Evaluate the patients knowledge about the medication and explain the use, action, dose and potential side effects of the medication

11. Ask the patient to lie on their side with the ear to be treated uppermost

12. Warm the drops to near body temperature by holding the drops in the palm of the hand for a few moments

13. Wash hands according to hand hygiene techniques and apply gloves and gown

14. Pull the cartilaginous part of the pinna backwards and upwards

15. If cerumen or drainage occludes the outermost part of the ear canal, wipe out gently with cotton tipped applicator

16. Allow the drops to fall in the direction of the external canal. The dropper should not touch the ear

17. Gently massage over tragus to help work in the drops

18. It may be necessary to temporarily place a gauze swab over the ear canal

19. Ask the patient to remain in this position for 2-3 minutes

20. Clean the equipment used according to manufacturer's recommendations and discard all disposable equipment gloves and apron in the appropriate/ clinical waste

21. Document the medication given and sign the prescription record

22. Decontaminate hands according to correct hand hygiene techniques

Source: Health Service Executive (2012). Guidelines for the administration of medications. HSE: Dublin.

11. Topical Medication Administration Guidelines

Equipment

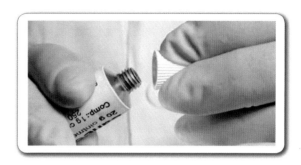

- Medication to be administered

- Medication record sheet

- Prescription chart

- Non-sterile gloves

- Apron

- Sterile topical swabs

- Applicators

- Dressing pack with sterile gloves (If aseptic technique required)

Procedure

1. Explain the procedure and gain informed consent

2. Decontaminate hands using correct hand hygiene techniques

3. Before administering any prescribed medication, check that is due and has not already been given

4. Carry out any required assessment such as pulse, BP, respiration, temperature

5. Check that the prescription is complete, correct and legible

6. Before administering any prescribed medication check the following

   - Correct patient

   - Correct medication

   - Correct dose

   - Date and time of administration

   - Diluent as appropriate

   - Validity of prescription

   - Signature of prescriber

   - Prescription is legible

If any of these pieces of information are missing, unclear or illegible then the nurse should not proceed with administration and should consult with the prescriber

7. Select the required medication and check the expiry date

8. Check the patients identity by confirming their name and date of birth or by checking their name band if necessary

9. Check the patients allergy status

10. Evaluate the patients knowledge about the medication and explain the use, action, dose and potential side effects of the medication

11. Assist the patient into the correct position and ensure privacy

12. Expose the area of skin that requires the topical medication and where necessary cover the patient with a towel or disposable sheet

13. Apply gloves and assess the condition of the skin, using aseptic techniques if the skin is broken

14. If the medication is to be rubbed into the skin, the preparation should be placed on a sterile topical swab

15. If the preparation causes staining advise the patient of this

16. Administer/ apply the topical medication as prescribed.

17. Apply a sterile dressing if required

18. Remove gloves and apron and dispose of waste appropriately

19. Document the medication given and sign the prescription record

20. Decontaminate hands according to correct hand hygiene techniques

Source: Health Service Executive (2012). Guidelines for the administration of medications. HSE: Dublin.

12. Vaginal Administration Guidelines

Equipment

- Pessary/ medication to be administered
- Prescription chart
- Non-sterile gloves
- Apron
- Topical swabs
- Lubricating Jelly
- Warm water
- Pen torch/ adequate light

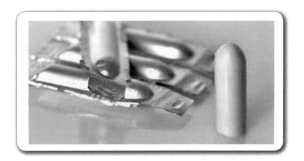

Procedure

1. Explain the procedure and gain informed consent

2. Decontaminate hands using correct hand hygiene techniques

3. Before administering any prescribed medication, check that is due and has not already been given

4. Carry out any required assessment such as pulse, BP, respiration, temperature

5. Check that the prescription is complete, correct and legible

6. Before administering any prescribed medication check the following

   - Correct patient
   - Correct medication
   - Correct dose
   - Date and time of administration
   - Diluent as appropriate
   - Validity of prescription
   - Signature of prescriber
   - Prescription is legible

If any of these pieces of information are missing, unclear or illegible then the nurse should not proceed with administration and should consult with the prescriber

7. Select the required medication/ pessary and check the expiry date

8. Check the patients identity by confirming their name and date of birth or by checking their name band if necessary

9. Check the patients allergy status

10. Evaluate the patients knowledge about the medication and explain the use, action, dose and potential side effects of the medication

11. Ensure privacy and assist the patient into the correct position: either left lateral with buttocks to the edge of the bed or supine with the knees drawn up and legs parted.

12. May require a light source, lamp or torch

13. Wash hands using correct hand hygiene techniques and apply gloves and apron

14. Clean the area with warm water if necessary

15. Remove the pessary from the wrapper and apply lubricating jelly to a topical swab and from the swab onto the pessary. Lubricate gloved index finger of dominant hand

16. With non-dominant gloved hand, gently retract labial folds to expose vaginal orifice

17. Insert the rounded end of the pessary along the posterior vaginal wall and into the top of the vagina

18. Wipe away any excess lubricating jelly from the patients vulva and or perineal area with a topical swab

19. Remove gloves and apron and dispose of waste appropriately

20. Document the medication given and sign the prescription record

21. Decontaminate hands according to correct hand hygiene techniques

Source: Health Service Executive (2012). Guidelines for the administration of medications. HSE: Dublin.

50. Intravenous Medication Administration Guidelines

1. Direct Injection, Bolus or Push

HSE (2013) Guidelines (Note 9.2) Administration by Direct Injection Bolus

9.2.1. Direct injection can be used when

the maximum serum concentration of the medicine is required to reach vital organs rapidly, e.g. adrenaline in the case of an emergency; the medicine cannot be further diluted for pharmacological or therapeutic reasons or does not require dilution. Too rapid administration can result in toxic levels and or anaphylactic type reaction. NB: this does not imply that this route is of quick administration in many cases it is 'slow IV injection' over 1-2 minutes depending on the medication.

9.2.2 This procedure may be carried out via any one of the following:

- An injection port attached to a Vascular Access Device
- An extension set

Equipment

- Patient's medication chart / Script
- Fluid Balance chart where appropriate
- Clinically clean tray or receiver with integrated sharps container
- PPE as required for specific medication
- Medications to be administered
- 21g needle(s) to ease reconstitution and drawing up, 23g for a glass ampoule
- Syringes of appropriate sizes for medication to be administered
- Sterile injection caps for syringes
- Medication additive labels
- Two 10ml syringes for flushes
- 0.9% Sodium Chloride 10 mls for injection or compatible solution
- Sterile 2% chlorahexidine gluconate in 70% alcohol swab, or sterile 70% isoprolol alcohol swab for cleaning injection site
- Latex non sterile disposable gloves for peripheral access, or sterile latex gloves for CVAD
- Sterile dressing pack if/ when accessing CVAD

Procedure:

1. Explain the procedure to the patient and obtain consent

2. Decontaminate hands using correct hand hygiene techniques

3. Before administering any prescribed medication check that it is due and has not been given already. Check the prescription is complete, correct and legible

4. Check the patient's allergy status

5. Check the intravenous cannula site for complications such as infiltration, phlebitis, redness or infection. Take appropriate action as necessary

6. Assemble all equipment, checking expiry dates and that the packaging is intact

7. Wash/ decontaminate hands and put on non-sterile latex disposable gloves

8. Maintain sterility of equipment that is in direct contact with the patient

9. Select and check the required medication against the medication chart/ prescription, checking packaging is intact. Inspect the container and contents for cracks, punctures, air bubbles, discoloration and haziness, crystalline or particulate matter

10. Check expiry dates

11. Check dosage/ calculate the correct dosage

12. Reconstitute using the correct diluent and volume

13. Prepare the flush solution. Draw up 0.9% Sodium Chloride for injection or compatible solution in two separate 10 ml syringes to use for flushing pre and post administration of medication to be administered. Apply a sterile cap to both syringes. Label each flush. Place the syringes/ flushes in a clinically clean receiver tray with the intravenous medication to be administered

14. Remove gloves and decontaminate hands

15. Identify patient. Check name, surname, date of birth, and medical record number if appropriate. In a community/ outpatient setting ascertain the patient's identity by verifying their name, date of birth and address. Where possible ask the patient to verbally confirm their details

16. Check the site and patency of the intravenous peripheral cannula

17. Wash/ decontaminate hands and put on gloves

18. Clean the administration site using a sterile 2% chlorahexidine gluconate in 70% alcohol swab. Allow to dry

19. Administer the flush slowly 5mls of 0.9% Sodium Chloride, to confirm patency of the cannula before administering medicinal preparations. Check that there is no resistance, pain, discomfort, swelling or leakage

20. Administer the intravenous medication slowly at the specified rate according to prescription

21. Observe the cannula insertion site for patency, swelling, leakage, infiltration or extravasation. Ask the patient to report any discomfort or pain

22. Stop the procedure if any adverse reaction occurs. Report same

23. After the medication has been administered, flush the cannula device with 5mls of 0.9% NACL (or other compatible solution for injection)

24. If more than one intravenous medication is to be administered, flush with sterile 0.9% sodium chloride or compatible solution between each administration

25. Immediately dispose of sharps in the sharps container and dispose of other waste in appropriate plastic bags

26. Decontaminate hands using correct hand hygiene techniques

27. Ensure the patient is comfortable

28. Document the administration appropriately in the notes

29. Record the fluid infused in the fluid balance chart where appropriate

Source: Health Service Executive (2013). National Policy for the Administration of Intravenous Medication by Registered Nurses and Midwives. HSE: Dublin.

2. Administration of Intermittent Infusion

HSE (2013) Guidelines (9.3) Administration of Intermittent Infusion

9.3.1 The delivery of an intermittent infusion can be by one of the following

9.3.1.1 Simultaneous infusion: the drug infusion is administered as a secondary infusion run concurrently with the primary infusion, attached to a lower secondary injection port.

9.3.1.2 Volume control set: the drug infusion is administered via a volume control set such as a burette.

9.3.1.3 Directly via the venous access device: the drug infusion is administered via an administration set connected to the venous access device. At the end of each infusion the drug container and administration set must be disconnected and discarded and the venous access device flushed as prescribed.

9.3.1.4 Some drugs that are administered by intermittent infusion are ready for infusion e.g., metronidazole. Other drugs require constitution and/or dilution prior to infusion. It is necessary to return to the patient at frequent intervals to ensure that the infusion is being delivered at the correct rate and to monitor for reactions or side effects.

Equipment

- Patient's medication Medication chart/ Script
- Fluid balance chart (if appropriate)
- Clinically clean tray or receiver with integrated sharps container
- PPE's as required for specific medication
- Medications to be administered
- Container/ bags of appropriate intravenous infusion fluids
- 21g needles to ease reconstitution and drawing up, 23 g for glass ampoules.
- Syringes (appropriate sizes)
- Intravenous administration set(s)
- Infusion device (syringe driver, infusomat where appropriate)
- Intravenous Infusion stand
- Sterile injection caps for syringes
- Medication additive labels
- Two 10ml syringes for flushes
- 0.9% sodium chloride10ml for injection (or compatible solution)

- Sterile 25 chlorahexidine gluconate in 70% alcohol swab or sterile 70% isopropyl alcohol swab for cleaning injection site
- Air inlet if appropriate
- Hypoallergenic tape
- Latex non sterile disposable gloves for peripheral access or sterile latex gloves for CVAD
- Cytotoxic spill kit (if necessary)

Procedure

1. Explain the procedure to the patient and obtain informed consent
2. Decontaminate hands using correct hand hygiene techniques
3. Before administering any prescribed medication check that it is due and has not been given already. Check the prescription is complete, correct and legible
4. Check the patient's allergy status
5. Check the intravenous cannula site for complications such as infiltration, phlebitis, redness or infection. Take appropriate action as necessary
6. Assemble all equipment, checking expiry dates and that the packaging is intact
7. Wash/ decontaminate hands and put on non-sterile latex disposable gloves
8. Select and check the required medication against the medication chart, checking packaging is intact
9. Check expiry dates
10. Calculate the correct dosage
11. Reconstitute using the correct diluent and volume
12. Inspect infusion fluid for discoloration, haziness, crystalline or particulate matter
13. Consider the following- compatibility of infusion fluids and additive/ stability of mixture over the prescribed time/ any special directions for dilution/ sensitivity to external factors such as light / any anticipated allergic reaction
14. Prepare the intravenous infusion and additive as described in the manufacturer's recommendations
15. Place the infusion bag on a flat surface. Remove any seal present on the inlet port

16. Clean the inlet port with a sterile 2% chlorahexidine gluconate in 70% alcohol swab or sterile 70% isopropolol alcohol swab and allow dry

17. Inject the medication using a new sterile needle into the infusion bag using an aseptic technique. A 23g or 24g needle should be used

18. Gently invert the infusion to avoid layering. Check for haziness, discoloration and particles

19. Complete and attach the medication additive label

20. Open the I.V administration set, and close the roller clamp. Attach the administration set aseptically to the intravenous infusion bag, being careful not to contaminate the inlet port. Take care not to puncture the bag

21. Prime the administration set with the infusion fluid. Hang it on the infusion stand

22. Check and prepare the flush solution. Draw up 5 mls of 0.9% sodium chloride for injection in two separate syringes. Apply a sterile cap to both syringes. Label each flush. Place in a clinically clean receiver or tray along with the I.V. medication to be administered

23. Remove gloves and decontaminate hands according to correct hand hygiene techniques

24. Identify patient. Check name, surname, date of birth, and medical record number if appropriate. In a community/ outpatient setting ascertain the patient's identity by verifying their name, date of birth and address. Where possible ask the patient to verbally confirm their details

25. Check the site and patency of the intravenous peripheral cannula

26. Decontaminate hands using correct hand hygiene techniques

27. Put on gloves

28. Clean the administration site using a sterile 2% chlorahexidine gluconate in 70% alcohol swab. Allow to dry

29. Gently administer the flush. Check that there is no resistance, pain, discomfort, swelling or leakage

30. Connect the infusion to the cannula device. Open the roller clamp and adjust the flow rate as prescribed

31. Monitor the flow rate and the intravenous site frequently for patency, swelling, leakage, infiltration or extravasation. Ask the patient to report any discomfort or pain

32. Stop the infusion if any adverse reaction occurs. Report same

33. When the infusion is complete, decontaminate hands and stop the infusion

34. Put on sterile gloves if appropriate

35. Disconnect the infusion set and flush the cannula device with 5mls of 0.9% NACL or other compatible solution for injection

36. Discard administration set after use

37. Immediately dispose of sharps in the sharps container and dispose of other waste in appropriate plastic bags

38. Decontaminate hands using correct hand hygiene techniques

39. Ensure the patient is comfortable

40. Document the administration appropriately in the notes

41. Record the fluid infused in the fluid balance chart where appropriate

Source: Health Service Executive (2013). National Policy for the Administration of Intravenous Medication by Registered Nurses and Midwives. HSE: Dublin.

51. Intravenous Hydrocortisone Administration Guidelines

Hydrocortisone Sodium Succinate (Solu-Cortef)

Action

Hydrocortisone is a short acting synthetic steroid with both glucocorticoid and mineralocorticoid properties that affect nearly all systems of the body. By inhibiting the formation, storage and release of histamine from mast cells, it reduces the effects of an allergic response. It also increases the body's response to circulating catecholamines.

Indications

Use of corticosteroids varies widely in different illnesses and different patients.

- Substitution therapy in the treatment of adrenal insufficiency
- Where high levels of hydrocortisone are required rapidly such as; Shock; Trauma or stress conditions
- Symptomatic relief of inflammatory conditions
- As an immunosuppressant

Contraindication

- Hypersensitivity to corticosteroids
- Tuberculosis
- Ocular herpes simplex
- Primary glaucoma
- Acute psychosis and psychoneurosis
- Systemic infection
- Peptic ulcer
- Osteoporosis

Warnings

Hydrocortisone sodium succinate injection should not be administered intrathecally or subconjunctivally. Toxic effects may result from withdrawal or from continued use of large doses. Hydrocortisone sodium succinate should be given with extreme caution in the presence of congestive heart failure; hypertension in patients with diabetes mellitus; chronic renal failure; uraemia and in elderly patients. Long-term steroid therapy can cause gastrointestinal bleeding, prolonged wound healing and suppression of the adrenocortical steroids.

Solu-Cortef should not be diluted or mixed with other solutions (possible incompatibilities).

Product should be inspected visually for particulate matter and discoloration prior to administration.

High dose corticosteroid therapy should be continued only until the patient's condition has stabilized- usually not beyond 48 to 72 hours. When high dose hydrocortisone therapy must be continued beyond 48–72 hours, hypernatremia may occur. Under such circumstances Solu-Cortef may be replaced with a corticoid such as methylprednisolone sodium succinate which causes little or no sodium retention.

Dosage requirements are variable and must be individualized on the basis of the disease under treatment and the response of the patient. After a favourable response is noted, the proper maintenance dosage should be determined by decreasing the initial drug dosage in small decrements at appropriate time intervals until the lowest dosage that maintains an adequate clinical response is reached. If after long-term therapy the drug is to be stopped, it is recommended that it be withdrawn gradually rather than abruptly.

Patient monitoring

- In high-dose therapy (which should not exceed 48 hours), watch closely for signs and symptoms of depression or psychotic episodes.
- Monitor blood pressure, weight, random blood sugars and electrolyte levels regularly.
- Assess blood glucose levels in diabetic patients. Expect to increase insulin or oral hypoglycemic dosage.
- Monitor patient's response during weaning from drug. Watch for adrenal crisis, which may occur if drug is discontinued too quickly.

Side effects and special precautions

Hydrocortisone sodium succinate may cause electrolyte disturbances, characterized by hypertension and oedema due to the retention of sodium and water and the increase in potassium excretion. Increased potassium excretion may cause hypokalaemic alkalosis. Increased susceptibility to infection (e.g. sepsis, fungal and viral) and delayed wound healing. Cardiac failure. Peptic ulcerations with haemorrhage and perforation. Glycosuria. Osteoporosis and spontaneous fractures. Increased appetite. Posterior subcapsular cataract. Atrophy of the adrenal cortex and acute adrenal insufficiency during prolonged treatment. Inhibition or arrest of growth in children. Cushing syndrome. Amenorrhoea. Behavioural disturbances, including mental and neurological disturbances. Intracranial hypertension. Thrombo-embolic complications. Lymphocytopaenia. Myopathy. Hyperglycaemia with accentuation or precipitation of the diabetic state. Insulin requirements of diabetic patients are increased. Infections may be masked by anti-inflammatory properties of Hydrocortisone sodium succinate. Hyperhydrosis and aseptic necrosis of bone may occur. Live vaccines should not be given to patients receiving high doses of Hydrocortisone sodium succinate. Patients receiving long courses of Hydrocortisone sodium succinate should be regularly checked for hypertension, glycosuria, hypokalaemia, gastric discomfort and mental changes. Sodium intake may have to be reduced and potassium supplements administered. Daily mass records may indicate fluid retention and back pain may signify osteoporosis. Children are at special risk from raised intracranial pressure. Infections should be treated as an emergency. Large doses should be given by infusion to prevent cardiovascular collapse. Concurrent administration of barbiturates, phenytoin or rifampicin may enhance the metabolism and reduce the effects of Hydrocortisone sodium succinate. Response to anti-coagulants may be reduced or enhanced. Concurrent administration of Hydrocortisone sodium succinate with potassium depleting diuretics may cause excessive potassium loss.

Storage

Store the un-reconstituted product at controlled room temperature (15 to 30°C). Store solution at controlled room temperature 15 to 30°C and protect from light. Use solution only if it is clear. Discard unused solutions after 3 days. The Act-O-Vial is a single dose vial and once reconstituted solution is used, any remaining portion should be discarded.

Administration of Hydrocortisone Sodium Succinate (Solu-Cortef)

Hydrocortisone sodium succinate is administered;

- **Intravenously as a bolus**
- **Intramuscularly**
- **Intravenous infusion**

The preferred method for initial use is by intravenous bolus injection
Following the initial period, consideration should be given to employing a longer acting injectable or oral preparation.

Dosage
100 to 500 mg Hydrocortisone succinate 3 to 4 times in 24 hours.

The dosage depends on the severity of the condition and the response.

52. Intravenous Bolus Therapy

Hydrocortisone Sodium Succinate (Solu-Cortef)

Therapy is initiated by administering Solu-Cortef intravenously as a bolus over a period of 30 seconds (e.g., 100 mg) to 10 minutes (e.g., 500 mg or more).

Prepare solution by aseptically adding not more than 2mls of Water for Injection or Sodium Chloride Injection to the contents of one vial.

Directions for using the Act-O-Vial System

1. Press down on plastic activator to force diluent into the lower compartment.
2. Gently agitate to effect solution.
3. Remove plastic tab covering centre of stopper.
4. Insert needle through centre of stopper until tip is just visible. Invert vial and withdraw dose.

Equipment

- Patient's medication chart
- Fluid Balance chart where appropriate
- Clinically clean tray or receiver with integrated sharps container
- PPE as required for specific medication
- Medication to be administered - Hydrocortisone Sodium Succinate (Solu-Cortef)
- 21g needle(s) to ease reconstitution and drawing up
- Syringes of appropriate sizes for medication to be administered
- Sterile injection caps for syringes
- Medication additive labels
- 10ml syringes x 2 for flushes
- 0.9% Sodium Chloride 10mls for injection or compatible solution
- Sterile 2% chlorahexidine gluconate in 70% alcohol swab, or sterile 70% isoprolol alcohol swab for cleaning injection site
- Latex non sterile disposable gloves for peripheral venous access, or sterile latex gloves for CVAD
- Sterile dressing pack when accessing CVAD

Procedure

1. Explain the procedure to the patient and obtain informed consent

2. Decontaminate hands using correct hand hygiene techniques

3. Before administering prescribed medication check that it is due and has not been given already. Check the prescription is complete, correct and legible.

4. Check the patient's allergy status

5. Check the intravenous cannula site for complications such as infiltration, phlebitis, redness or infection. Take appropriate action as necessary

6. Assemble all equipment, checking expiry dates and that the packaging is intact.

7. Wash/ decontaminate hands and put on non-sterile latex disposable gloves

8. Maintain sterility of equipment that is in direct contact with the patient

9. Select and check the required medication against the medication chart/ prescription, checking packaging is intact. Inspect the container and contents for cracks, punctures, air bubbles, discoloration and haziness, crystalline or particulate matter

10. Check expiry dates

11. Check dosage/ calculate the correct dosage

12. Reconstitute using the correct diluent and volume

13. Prepare the flush solution. Draw up 0.9% Sodium Chloride for injection or compatible solution in two separate 10 ml syringes to use for flushing pre and post administration of medication to be administered. Apply a sterile cap to both syringes. Label each flush. Place the syringes/ flushes in a clinically clean receiver tray with the intravenous medication to be administered

14. Remove gloves and decontaminate hands

15. Identify patient. Check name, surname, date of birth, and medical record number if appropriate. In a community/ outpatient setting ascertain the patient's identity by verifying their name, date of birth and address. Where possible ask the patient to verbally confirm their details

16. Check the site and patency of the intravenous peripheral cannula

17. Decontaminate hands using correct hand hygiene techniques

18. Put on gloves

19. Clean the administration site using a sterile 2% chlorahexidine gluconate in 70% alcohol swab. Allow to dry

20. Administer the flush slowly 5mls of 0.9% Sodium Chloride (or other compatible solution for injection), to confirm patency of the cannula before administering medicinal preparations. Check there is no resistance, pain, discomfort, swelling or leakage

21. Administer the intravenous medication slowly at the specified rate according to prescription

22. Observe the cannula insertion site for patency, swelling, leakage, infiltration or extravasation. Ask the patient to report any discomfort or pain

23. Stop the procedure if any adverse reaction occurs. Report same

24. After the medication has been administered, flush the cannula device with 5mls of 0.9% NACL (or other compatible solution for injection)

25. If more than one intravenous medication is to be administered, flush with sterile 0.9% sodium chloride or compatible solution between each administration

26. Immediately dispose of sharps in the sharps container and dispose of other waste in appropriate plastic bags

27. Decontaminate hands using correct hand hygiene techniques

28. Ensure the patient is comfortable

29. Document the administration appropriately in the notes

30. Record the fluid infused in the fluid balance chart where appropriate.

53. Intravenous Infusion of Hydrocortisone

Intravenous Infusion Therapy (Solu-Cortef)

Prepare solution by adding not more than 2mls of Water for Injection to the vial; this solution may then be added to 100mls to 1000mls of the following: 5% dextrose in water (or isotonic saline solution or 5% dextrose in isotonic saline solution if patient is not on sodium restriction).

- **The 100 mg solution may be added to 100 to 1000 mls of 5%** Dextrose in Water (or isotonic saline solution or 5% dextrose in isotonic saline solution if patient is not on sodium restriction).

- **The 250 mg solution may be added to 250 to 1000 mls of 5%** Dextrose in Water (or isotonic saline solution or 5% dextrose in isotonic saline solution if patient is not on sodium restriction).

- **The 500 mg solution may be added to 500 to 1000 mls of 5%** Dextrose in Water (or isotonic saline solution or 5% dextrose in isotonic saline solution if patient is not on sodium restriction).

- **The 1000 mg solution may be added to 1000 mls of 5%** Dextrose in Water (or isotonic saline solution or 5% dextrose in isotonic saline solution if patient is not on sodium restriction).

In cases, where administration of a small volume of fluid is desirable, 100 mg to 3000 mg of Solu-Cortef may be added to 50 mls of the above diluents. The resulting solutions are stable for at least 4 hours and may be administered either directly or by IV piggy back.

Equipment

- Medication chart/ prescription
- Fluid balance chart (if appropriate)
- Clinically clean tray or receiver with integrated sharps container
- PPE's as required for specific medication
- Medication to be administered- Hydrocortisone Sodium Succinate (Solu-Cortef)
- Container/ bags of appropriate intravenous infusion fluids
- 21g needles to ease reconstitution and drawing up
- Syringes (appropriate sizes)
- Intravenous administration set.

- Infusion device (syringe driver, infusomat where appropriate)
- Intravenous Infusion stand
- Sterile injection caps for syringes
- Medication additive labels
- 10ml syringes x 2 for flushes
- 0.9% sodium chloride10ml for injection (or compatible solution)
- Sterile 25 chlorahexidine gluconate in 70% alcohol swab or sterile 70% isopropyl alcohol swab for cleaning injection site
- Air inlet if appropriate
- Hypoallergenic tape
- Latex non sterile disposable gloves for peripheral access or sterile latex gloves for CVAD

Procedure

1. Explain the procedure to the patient and obtain informed consent
2. Decontaminate hands using correct hand hygiene techniques
3. Before administering prescribed medication check that it is due and has not been given already. Check the prescription is complete, correct and legible
4. Check the patient's allergy status
5. Check the intravenous cannula site for complications such as infiltration, phlebitis, redness or infection. Take appropriate action as necessary
6. Assemble all equipment, checking expiry dates and that the packaging is intact.
7. Decontaminate hands and put on non-sterile latex disposable gloves
8. Select and check the required medication against the medication chart, checking packaging is intact
9. Check expiry dates
10. Calculate the correct dosage
11. Reconstitute using the correct diluent and volume
12. Inspect infusion fluid for discoloration, haziness, crystalline or particulate matter
13. Consider the following- compatibility of infusion fluids and additive/ stability of mixture over the prescribed time/ any special directions for dilution/ sensitivity to external factors such as light / any anticipated allergic reaction

14. Prepare the intravenous infusion and additive as described in the manufacturer's recommendations

15. Place the infusion bag on a flat surface. Remove any seal present on the inlet port

16. Clean the inlet port with a sterile 2% chlorahexidine gluconate in 70% alcohol swab or sterile 70% isopropolol alcohol swab and allow dry

17. Inject the medication using a new sterile needle into the infusion bag using an aseptic technique. A 23g or 24g needle should be used

18. Gently invert the infusion to avoid layering. Check for haziness, discoloration and particles

19. Complete and attach the medication additive label

20. Open the I.V administration set, and close the roller clamp. Attach the administration set aseptically to the intravenous infusion bag, being careful not to contaminate the inlet port. Take care not to puncture the bag

21. Prime the administration set with the infusion fluid. Hang it on the infusion stand

22. Check and prepare the flush solution. Draw up 5mls of 0.9% sodium chloride for injection (or compatible solution) in two separate syringes. Apply a sterile cap to both syringes. Label each flush. Place in a clinically clean receiver or tray along with the I.V. medication to be administered

23. Remove gloves and clean hands according to correct hand hygiene techniques

24. Identify patient. Check name, surname, date of birth, and medical record number if appropriate. In a community/ outpatient setting ascertain the patient's identity by verifying their name, date of birth and address. Where possible ask the patient to verbally confirm their details

25. Check the site and patency of the intravenous peripheral cannula

26. Decontaminate hands according to correct hand hygiene techniques. Put on gloves

27. Clean the administration site using a sterile 2% chlorahexidine gluconate in 70% alcohol swab. Allow to dry

28. Gently administer the flush. Check that there is no resistance, pain, discomfort, swelling or leakage

29. Connect the infusion to the cannula device. Open the roller clamp and adjust the flow rate as prescribed

30. Note: Alternatively if using infusion monitoring device, (syringe driver, infusomat) use according to manufacturer's instructions. Set dose, rate and volume appropriately

31. Monitor the flow rate and the intravenous site frequently for patency, swelling, leakage, infiltration or extravasation. Ask the patient to report any discomfort/ pain

32. Stop the infusion if any adverse reaction occurs. Report same

33. When the infusion is complete, decontaminate hands and stop the infusion

34. Put on sterile gloves if appropriate

35. Disconnect the infusion set and flush the cannula device with 5mls of 0.9% NACL or other compatible solution for injection

36. Discard administration set after use

37. Immediately dispose of sharps in the sharps container and dispose of other waste in appropriate plastic bags

38. Decontaminate hands using correct hand hygiene techniques

39. Ensure the patient is comfortable

40. Document the administration appropriately in the notes

41. Record the fluid infused in the fluid balance chart where appropriate

References

Health Service Executive (2013). National Policy for the Administration of Intravenous Medication by Registered Nurses and Midwives. HSE: Dublin.

St Luke's Hospital (2011). Policy for the Administration of Intravenous Medicinal Preparations by Nursing and Midwifery Staff; St Luke's Hospital. Kilkenny, Ireland.

54. Central Venous Access Devices Hickman Catheters and PICC Lines

There are many different types of central lines but the three most commonly used types of Central Venous Access Devices (CVAD's) are

- Hickmann Skin Tunnelled Catheters
- PICC - Peripherally Inserted Central Catheters
- Tunnelled Implanted Ports (Port-a-Cath)

Central venous access devices (CVAD's) are permitted to be used for:

1. Blood sampling
2. Administration of all IV therapies and treatments
3. Blood product administration
4. Dye studies

Hickmann Skin Tunnelled Catheters

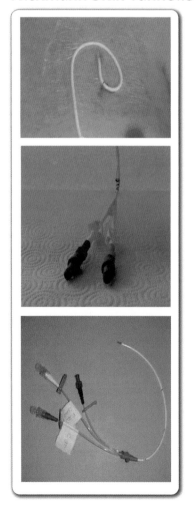

The Hickman Catheter is a large bore silicon catheter. When inserted one end of the catheter is introduced into a vein (usually the cephalic, subclavian, internal or external jugular vein) with the catheter tip located in the lower third of the superior vena cava. The other end is tunnelled under the skin and pulled through so that the tunnel provides a distance between the entry and exit site. The distance between the entry and exit site helps reduce the risk of bacteria from the skin contaminating the bloodstream. These devices have a dacron cuff attached to the portion of catheter that is tunnelled under the skin. The patient's tissue granulates around this cuff which both helps hold the catheter in place and also acts as a mechanical barrier to ascending bacteria. Tunnelled CVAD's are available in single, double and triple lumen catheters. These catheters are surgically inserted and can be selected for long term vascular access e.g. chemotherapy and TPN (over 30 days) and provide stable anchorage in patients who require long term IV therapy.

Peripherally inserted Central Catheters (PICC) and Midline Catheters

The PICC is a fine bore catheter which is inserted into a peripheral vein (usually the basilic or cephalic vein) and threaded towards the heart with its tip located in the lower third of the superior vena cava. These catheters can usually be inserted at the patient's bedside and can provide venous access for up to a year or more. When frequent and continuous access is necessary which is likely to exceed 6 days, a PICC or tunnelled CVAD is preferable. (Midline catheters provide vascular access in a large peripheral vein without entering the central venous circulation). Both lines are associated with lower rates of phlebitis and infection compared with peripheral venous catheters.

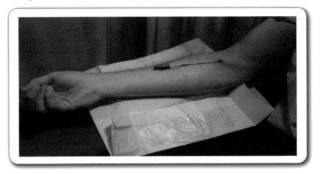

Tunnelled Implanted Ports (Port-a-Cath)

The implantable port differs from other CVAD's because it has no external parts. The port sits under the patient's skin on the chest wall, lower rib cage or anticubital area. It is made up of a portal body and attached to a silicon catheter which sits in the lower third of the superior vena cava. It has a self-sealing septum which is accessed through intact skin and again it can be used for long term vascular access (over 30 days).These devices have the lowest rates of catheter related blood stream infections

55. Dressings for Hickman Catheters and PICC Lines

Inspection/Assessment

1. Before inspection of all CVAD's, decontaminate hands and wrists using correct hand hygiene techniques

2. To help prevent catheter related infection it is essential to detect problems at the earliest opportunity. The insertion site should be visibly inspected

3. Always change the dressing if it becomes soiled, loosened or damp

4. Otherwise change dressings every 7 days including observing Manufacturer's recommendations

5. If tubigrip/tubinet is in place on PICC lines roll down with decontaminated hands to inspect site.

6. If a gauze dressing is used this will require dressing daily. A gauze dressing should be replaced by a transparent dressing as soon as possible

7. PICC lines post insertion will have a small piece of sterile gauze over the insertion site which acts as a wick. This will help absorb any exudate from the insertion site and should be left in place for 24 hours only, i.e. until the first dressing change on day after line insertion.

Recommended dressings

1. A sterile transparent self-adhesive semi permeable dressing such as the IV 3000 is preferable because it allows continuous undisturbed visual inspection of the catheter site, requires less frequent changing and allows the patient to shower and bathe without saturating the dressing

2. If the site is oozing/bleeding, if the patient is diaphoretic or unable to tolerate a semi permeable transparent dressing a sterile gauze dressing is preferable, though this will require changing daily when inspecting the site, or more frequently if it becomes loose, damp or soiled

3. Tunnelled CVAD's that are well healed may not require dressings

4. CVAD's should be assessed at least twice a day. All observations and nursing actions taken during the care of CVAD's must be documented in the patient's nursing notes

5. Patient education regarding dressing care and maintenance should be documented in the patient's nursing notes

6. Vascular access site care shall be performed using aseptic non-touch technique and observing standard precautions

7. Ensure antiseptics used for catheter site care are compatible with the catheter material. Refer to manufacturer's instructions and only use recommended antiseptics

Equipment for dressing change

- Dressing trolley – disinfect a visibly clean trolley using large 70% alcohol wipe.
- Sterile dressing pack
- Extra sterile gauze squares as necessary
- Antiseptic solution for skin disinfection e.g. chlorhexidine gluconate 2% and isopropyl alcohol 70%.
- Single patient use application solution of 2% chlorhexidine gluconate in isopropyl alcohol 70% wipes.
- Semi permeable transparent dressing e.g. IV 3000
- Sterile latex gloves
- Individually wrapped needle free connector(s)
- Steri-strips for PICC lines only
- Sterile impervious sheet if not included in dressing pack

Check all equipment/preparations

Do not use if packaging is contaminated or damaged or if expiry date is exceeded. With each procedure adhere to standard precautions and using appropriate PPE e.g. gloves, goggles, apron as required

Procedure for dressing change

1. Identify the patient. Check patient's name, date of birth and hospital number against the patient's identification band if the patient is an inpatient. In an outpatient situation, ascertain the patient's identity by verifying the name, date of birth and address

2. Provide the patient with privacy. Explain the procedure to the patient and give him/her the opportunity to voice any concerns, express any preferences or ask any questions. Where possible informed verbal consent must be obtained before beginning the procedure

3. Check if the patient has any known allergies to skin preparations or adhesive material

4. Decontaminate hands and wrists using correct hand hygiene techniques

5. Open dressing pack taking care only to touch the corners, i.e. do not touch the inside of the sterile field and open all of the above equipment aseptically onto the sterile field

6. Wearing non sterile gloves, remove old dressing(s). Remove gauze wick and steri-strips from PICC line if present. Place dressings directly in small health care risk bag. Remove gloves, place in small health care risk bag and disinfect hands and wrists by applying an alcohol based hand-rub

7. Visually inspect entry/exit sites for signs of infection exudate, redness, oozing and tracking

8. Discuss observations with patient and check if they are experiencing any symptoms e.g. pain, swelling or tenderness at exit site and/or entry site

9. Put on sterile gloves

10. With a Hickman line ensure the dacron cuff is not visible at exit site. If it is, cover site with sterile dressing and inform the medical team.

11. Request the patient or a staff member to lift catheter line. Place the sterile impervious sheet under the catheter line and needle free connector

12. Clean exit site in a circular outward direction with a single patient use application solution of 2% chlorhexidine gluconate and 70% isopropyl alcohol

13. Allow the solution to air dry to enable the disinfection process to be completed

Direction in which to clean exit site

1. To clean down the line: Immobilise the line by holding it with a piece of dry sterile gauze at the exit site with one hand. Clean down the line from exit site to just above the bung if single lumen catheter, and to 'the junction' if more than one lumen catheter using an individually wrapped large 2% chlorhexidine gluconate in 70% isopropyl wipe. Use each wipe once and discard

2. Allow the solution to air dry to enable the disinfection process to be completed

3. For more than single lumen CVAD's clean each lumen separately

4. Clean from the top of the needle free connector up to 'the junction' using an individually wrapped large 2% chlorhexidine gluconate in 70% isopropyl wipe. Use each wipe once and discard

5. Immobilise the needle free connector by holding it with a piece of dry sterile gauze in one hand

6. Clean around the junction area with the individually wrapped large 2% chlorhexidine gluconate in 70% isopropyl wipe. Use each wipe once and discard

7. Allow the solution to air dry to enable the disinfection process to be completed

8. Clean needle free connector using an individually wrapped large 2% chlorhexidine gluconate in 70% isopropyl wipe. Apply wipe firmly and rotate five times over the silicone surface and associated rim of the device and allow the solution to air dry. Discard used wipe

9. Finally loop the Hickman line under a semi permeable transparent dressing e.g. IV 3000 dressing to prevent trauma to the line which could be caused by accidental pulling of the catheter

10. With PICC lines apply new sterile steri-strips before applying a semi permeable transparent dressing e.g. IV 3000 dressing. A loose bandage e.g. Tubigrip / tubinet can be used over the PICC line dressing to help secure and protect it. Replace at each dressing change or more frequently if required

11. Remove gloves and any other PPE and dispose in appropriate waste bag

12. Decontaminate hands using correct hand hygiene technique

13. Fold up sterile field and dispose into appropriate health care risk waste bag. Decontaminate trolley/ clinical field and wash hands

References
University Hospital Waterford (2018). Guidelines for the Care and Maintenance of Long Term Central Venous Access Devices (CVAD's). UHW. Waterford

56. Flushing Tunnelled CVAD's

Hickman Lines and PICC Lines

1. All CVAD's must be checked for patency prior to each manipulation, e.g. blood sampling and/or the infusion of intravenous therapies. All CVAD's must be flushed after each manipulation of the line and once weekly if line not in use to maintain patency

2. A size 10ml or greater sterile leur lock syringe should only be used on all types of CVAD's to prevent damage/fracture to the line

3. Following the weekly flushing it will be necessary to routinely change the needle free connector(s) in accordance with manufacturer's instructions

4. It is necessary to continuously refer to manufacturer's instructions to ensure that maximum period of use of the device(s) has not altered

The flushing of these lines is to help prevent vascular thrombosis, microbial adherence and catheter related blood stream infection

Equipment

- Dressing trolley – disinfect a visibly clean trolley using large 70% alcohol wipe

- Sterile dressing pack

- Extra sterile gauze squares as needed

- Single patient use application solution of 2% chlorhexidine gluconate in isopropyl alcohol 70% wipes

- Sterile gloves

- Individually wrapped needle free connector(s)

- 10 ml sterile leur lock syringes and sterile needles

- 10mls 0.9% sodium chloride for injection for each lumen

- Heparin sodium 10iu /ml IV flush solution eg. Heplock. for each Hickman lumen

- Heparin sodium 100iu/ml IV flush solution e.g. Heprinse for each PICC lumen

- Sterile impervious sheet if not included in dressing pack

- Sharps container

Check all equipment/preparations

Do not use if packaging is contaminated or damaged or if expiry date is exceeded. With each procedure adhere to standard precautions and using appropriate PPE e.g. gloves, goggles, apron as required

Procedure

1. Refer to first four points of section on Procedure for Dressing Change

2. Decontaminate hands using correct hand hygiene techniques

3. Open dressing pack taking care only to touch the corners i.e. do not touch the inside of the sterile field, and open all of the above sterile equipment aseptically onto the sterile field

4. Check the 0.9% sodium chloride and heparin solutions with a second registered nurse/medical practitioner

5. Visually inspect entry/exit sites for signs of infection i.e. exudate, redness, oozing, tracking

6. Discuss observations with patient and check if they are experiencing any symptoms e.g. pain, swelling or tenderness at exit site and/or entry site

7. Disinfect hands and wrists by applying an alcohol based hand-rub as described above and put on sterile gloves

8. With a Hickman line ensure the dacron cuff is not visible at exit site. If it is cover site with a sterile dressing and inform the medical team

9. If there are signs of infection present inform the medical team

10. Aseptically draw up the 0.9% sodium chloride and heparinised solutions from the vial(s). Remove needle and dispose directly into sharps container

11. Place syringe(s) in sterile dish of dressing pack

12. Request the patient or a staff member to lift catheter line. Place the sterile impervious sheet under the catheter line and needle free connector(s)

Follow the procedure below for each lumen of Hickman catheter

13. Clean needle free connector using an individually wrapped large 2% chlorhexidine gluconate in 70% isopropyl wipe. Apply wipe firmly and rotate five times over the silicone surface and associated rim of the device and allow the solution to air dry. Discard used wipe

14. Attach 10ml sterile leur lock syringe to bung and drawback to check for blood return

15. Should no blood return refer to Section on Complications of CVAD's re Partial or Complete Catheter Occlusion

16. Once blood return is present instill 10mls of 0.9% sodium chloride followed by 5mls of heparin sodium 10iu/ml IV flush solution as prescribed e.g. Heplock, clamping the catheter as the last ½ml is infusing to ensure that positive pressure is maintained, thus preventing backflow and clotting of blood. Always follow manufacturer's instructions

17. Remove needle free connector and clean open end of lumen with an individually wrapped large 2% chlorhexidine gluconate in 70% isopropyl wipe. Apply the wipe firmly and rotate five times over the silicone surface and associated rim of the devise and allow the solution to air dry prior to attaching a new individually wrapped needle free connector. Discard used wipe

18. Remove gloves and any other PPE and dispose in appropriate waste bag. Wash hands as above. Fold up sterile field and dispose into appropriate health care risk waste bag. Decontaminate trolley/ clinical field and wash hands

For PICC Lines

Follow procedure as above and once blood return is present instil into each lumen 10mls of 0.9% sodium chloride followed by 4mls of heparin sodium 100iu/ml IV flush solution as prescribed e.g. Heprinse, again clamping the catheter as the last ½ml is infusing to ensure that positive pressure is maintained, thus preventing backflow and clotting of blood

19. Remove needle free connector and clean open end of lumen with an individually wrapped large 2% chlorhexidine gluconate in 70% isopropyl wipe. Apply the wipe firmly and rotate five times over the silicone surface and associated rim of the devise and allow the solution to air dry prior to attaching a new individually wrapped needle free connector. Discard used wipe

20. Remove gloves and any other PPE and dispose in appropriate waste bag. Wash hands as above. Fold up sterile field and dispose into appropriate health care risk waste bag. Decontaminate trolley/ clinical field and clean hands according to correct hand hygiene techniques

References

National Health Service (2010). Guidelines for the Care and Maintenance of Central Venous Access Devices. Sutton and Merton NHS Trust: England.

Health Service Executive (2010). Guidelines for the Care and Maintenance of Long Term Central Venous Access Devices (CVAD's) in University Hospital Waterford excluding Dialysis Lines. UHW: Waterford.

University Hospital Waterford (2018). Guidelines for the Care and Maintenance of Long Term Central Venous Access Devices (CVAD's). UHW: Waterford.

57. Infusing via Tunnelled CVAD's Hickman and PICC Lines

Equipment

- Dressing trolley – disinfect a visibly clean trolley using large 70% alcohol wipe

- Sterile dressing pack

- Single patient use application solution of 2% chlorhexidine gluconate in isopropyl alcohol 70% wipes

- Medications to be administered/ Prescription or Medication chart

- Correct dilutants and volume for reconstitution (e.g. Sterile Water for Injection)

- Required fluids e.g. 50 or 100 ml bag(s) of NACL

- Appropriate syringes and needles for preparing and adding medication to fluids for infusion

- Required flush solutions (NACL/ Heparin if prescribed)

- Sterile caps

- Infusion (Giving) set(s)

- Pump (if required)

- Sterile gloves

- 10ml sterile leur lock syringe

- Sterile impervious sheet if not included in dressing pack

- Sharps container

Check all equipment/preparations

Do not use if packaging is contaminated or damaged or if expiry date is exceeded. With each procedure adhere to standard precautions and using appropriate PPE e.g. gloves, goggles, apron as required

Procedure

General principles for preparing IV infusions

1. Assemble all equipment, checking expiry dates and that the packaging is intact

2. Wash/ decontaminate hands and put on non-sterile latex disposable gloves

3. Select and check the required medication against the medication chart, checking packaging is intact

4. Check expiry dates

5. Calculate the correct dosage

6. Reconstitute using the correct diluent and volume

7. Inspect infusion fluid for discoloration, haziness, crystalline or particulate matter

8. Consider the following- compatibility of infusion fluids and additive/ stability of mixture over the prescribed time/ any special directions for dilution/ sensitivity to external factors such as light / any anticipated allergic reaction

9. Prepare the intravenous infusion and additive as described in the manufacturer's recommendations

10. Place the infusion bag on a flat surface. Remove any seal present on the inlet port

11. Clean the inlet port with a sterile 2% chlorahexidine gluconate in 70% alcohol swab or sterile 70% isopropolol alcohol swab and allow dry

12. Inject the medication using a new sterile needle into the infusion bag using an aseptic technique. A 23g or 24g needle should be used

13. Gently invert the infusion to avoid layering. Check for haziness, discoloration and particles

14. Complete and attach the medication additive label

15. Open the I.V administration set, and close the roller clamp. Attach the administration set aseptically to the intravenous infusion bag, being careful not to contaminate the inlet port. Take care not to puncture the bag

16. Prime the administration set with the infusion fluid. Hang it on the infusion stand

17. Check and prepare the flush solutions. Label each flush and apply sterile cap

18. Place in a clinically clean receiver or tray along with the I.V. medication to be administered

19. Remove gloves and wash/ decontaminate hands

Refer to first four points on section on Procedure for Dressing Change

1. Decontaminate hands according to correct hand hygiene techniques

2. Open dressing pack taking care only to touch the corners i.e. do not touch the inside of the sterile field, and open all of the above sterile equipment aseptically onto the sterile field

3. Visually inspect entry/exit sites for signs of infection i.e. exudate/redness/oozing and/or tracking

4. Discuss observations with patient and check if they are experiencing any symptoms e.g. pain, swelling or tenderness at exit site and/or entry site

5. Disinfect hands and wrists by applying an alcohol based hand rub and put on sterile gloves

6. With a Hickman line ensure the dacron cuff is not visible at exit site. If it is, cover site with sterile dressing and inform the medical team

7. If there are signs of infection present refer to medical team

8. Request the patient or a staff member to lift catheter line. Place the sterile impervious sheet under the catheter line and needle free connector(s)

9. Clean needle free connector using an individually wrapped large 2% chlorhexidine gluconate in 70% isopropyl wipe. Apply the wipe firmly and rotate through five times over the silicone surface and associated rim of the devise and allow the solution to air dry. Discard used wipe

10. Attach 10ml sterile leur lock syringe to needle free connector and drawback to check for blood return

11. Should no blood return refer to Section on Complications of CVAD's re Partial or Complete Catheter Occlusion

12. Once blood return is present (refer to flushing guidelines and individual patients prescribed flush requirements) then connect aseptically the prescribed infusion (via pump if required) to the CVAD -adhering to correct rate, volume and time

13. Dispose of waste into appropriate health care risk waste bags and sharps bin

14. Remove gloves. Decontaminate hands according to correct hand hygiene techniques

References

National Health Service (2010). Guidelines for the Care and Maintenance of Central Venous Access Devices. Sutton and Merton NHS Trust: England.

Health Service Executive (2010). Guidelines for the Care and Maintenance of Long Term Central Venous Access Devices (CVAD's) in University Hospital Waterford excluding Dialysis Lines. UHW: Waterford.

University Hospital Waterford (2018). Guidelines for the Care and Maintenance of Long Term Central Venous Access Devices (CVAD's). UHW: Waterford.

Note: Refer to main policy guidelines & procedures folder for preparation and administration of each individual prescribed IV medication/ infusion to be administered

58. Disconnection of Infusions from Tunnelled CVAD's

Hickman Lines and PICC Lines

With each procedure adhere to standard precautions and using appropriate PPE e.g. gloves, goggles, apron as required.

Procedure

1. Refer to first four points of section on Procedure for Dressing Change

2. Decontaminate hands according to correct hand hygiene techniques

3. Visually inspect entry/exit sites for signs of infection i.e. exudate, redness, oozing, tracking

4. Discuss observations with patient and check if they are experiencing any symptoms e.g. pain, swelling or tenderness at exit site and/or entry site

5. With a Hickman line ensure the dacron cuff is not visible at exit site. If it is, turn off infusion and clamp catheter lumen. Decontaminate hands and wrists by applying an alcohol based hand rub. Put on sterile gloves and cover site with sterile dressing before informing the medical team

6. Turn off infusion, clamp catheter lumen, disconnect infusion and dispose of giving set and infusion bag in appropriate health care waste bags and sharps bin

7. To complete flushing of lumen refer to the section on Equipment and Procedure for Flushing CVAD's (Hickman Lines & PICC Lines) and the patient's prescription

Source: University Hospital Waterford (2018). Guidelines for the Care and Maintenance of Long Term Central Venous Access Devices (CVAD's). UHW. Waterford.

59. Complications of CVAD's

Hickman and PICC Lines

1. Infection

This is the most frequent complication associated with CVAD's. Infection can occur within the catheter, at the exit site or skin tunnel. Patient's skin and healthcare workers hands are the main sources of pathogens

Risk factors include

- Poor aseptic technique
- Length of time the catheter is in situ
- Patients underlying condition
- Number of lumens
- Insufficient patient and staff education
- Administration of TPN
- To-and-fro' motion of the catheter

Signs and Symptoms of infection

- Pyrexia
- Pain/tenderness at site
- Redness
- Erythema
- Exudate may/may not be present
- Tracking may/may not be present
- Swelling/oedema

What to do if infection suspected

- Contact the medical practitioner
- Obtain a swab for culture and sensitivity from entry/exit site
- Two sets of blood cultures should be taken separately from each lumen of the CVAD and peripherally (both aerobic and anaerobic)
- Document vital signs i.e. Temperature, pulse, blood pressure and respiration rate

To help reduce the risk of infection:

1. Strict handwashing regime should be followed at all times
2. Appropriate use of PPE
3. Aseptic technique for each procedure
4. Monitor the catheter and catheter site care to help minimise infection
5. Minimise the number of times that the line is manipulated/infusions are disconnected. If a line is disconnected the infusion set should be discarded and a new one started
6. Infusions of TPN should be infused undisturbed except when absolutely necessary e.g. when taking blood cultures
7. Staff, patients and carers involved in looking after CVAD's should receive continuous and ongoing education
8. Change intravenous administration sets as per manufacturer's instructions

2. Catheter Malposition

A chest x-ray is performed after the insertion of a CVAD to verify its position. A CVAD may become mal-positioned not only as a result of the insertion procedure but also by spontaneous migration or following a repair procedure.

3. Partial or complete catheter occlusions

A CVAD may become occluded or sluggish and unable to aspirate blood from it for a number of reasons:

3.1 Thrombosis

Symptoms of central vein thrombus around the catheter tip include oedema of the arm, shoulder or neck, distended veins and collateral circulation. The chest x-ray should be checked to confirm that the catheter tip lies within the superior vena cava.

3.2 Pinch off syndrome

This occurs when the CVAD is compressed between the clavicle and the first rib, causing intermittent occlusion during infusion and withdrawal. Prolonged pinch off syndrome can cause the catheter to rupture and migrate through the blood vessels and into the heart. Pinch off syndrome can be diagnosed by chest x-ray or dye studies.

3.3 Fibrin Sheath Formation

Fibrin deposition can occur at the end of the CVAD or along the length of the CVAD and wall of the vein. When it is located around the tip of the catheter it can be difficult to aspirate blood from the line but usually infusing fluids is not a problem. But resistance may be felt during infusing or there may be a marked reduction in the rate at which fluids can be infused. This will result in occlusion or thrombus formation if left unresolved.

3.4 Precipitation of Medication

Precipitation is often the result of inadequate flushing between the administration of incompatible drugs/solutions which can occur suddenly and can occlude the CVAD.

1. If there is no blood returned from a CVAD after checking that there is no external occlusion, such as a kinked line, a bra strap or the clamp is closed, ask the patient to cough, breathe deeply and/or change position and aspirate again

2. If unsuccessful, inject 1-2mls of normal saline or a heparin sodium solution using a 10ml sterile leur lock syringe, without using excessive force and aspirate again

3. If unsuccessful request a chest x-ray and have same reviewed by a medical practitioner. If indicated, dye studies may then be ordered

4. Further management: the use of Urokinase if recommended by the medical team

4. Air embolus

This is a potentially preventable complication of CVAD placement and removal. It is the result of air entering the venous circulation and travelling to the pulmonary vein. The risk of it occurring can be minimised by placing the patient in the Trendelenburg position or in the case of PICC insertions, by insuring that the patient's arm is kept below the level of the heart

5. Pneumothorax

This occurs if air enters the space between the pleural lining and the lung. All tunnelled CVAD's require a chest x-ray post insertion to check for pneumothorax

6. Haemothorax

This can be a result of puncturing the subclavian vein or artery during insertion and causes blood to leak into the pleural cavity

7. Arterial Puncture

This will occur if an artery is cannulated or punctured during the insertion procedure and is recognisable by the spurting of bright red blood into the syringe or through the cannula /introducer

8. Nerve Injury

The ulna and median nerves can be damaged during PICC insertion if they accidentally come in contact with the cannula/introducer. Similarly damage to the radial cords of the brachial plexus can also result from subclavian placements of other types of CVAD

9. Atrial Fibrillation

This can occur if the catheter extends beyond the superior vena cava and into the right atrium

10. Catheter Fracture

Rupture of a CVAD can be prevented by ensuring that high-pressure methods of drug/fluid administration are avoided. Catheter fracture can be caused by excessive syringe pressure when flushing a catheter. A 10ml sterile leur lock syringe is the smallest size recommended for use with CVAD's. Pinch off syndrome as explained in section 3.2 can also cause catheter fracture. If a CVAD fractures, this can cause infiltration or extravasation of fluids / medication into the surrounding tissue at the fracture site. It is important to ensure that the catheter is secured to the patients skin when connected to an infusion otherwise the device can twist. The increasing stress from the twisting can result in damage and possibly a fracture of the CVAD

11. Catheter Fracture Repair

Only personnel who are experienced in this procedure should carry out the repair and the procedure must be carried out aseptically. The manufacturers of the various CVAD's provide repair kits for their specific products together with comprehensive instructions to repair the external portion of single, double and triple lumen Hickman and PICC lines

Repair kits contain; a catheter section with adaptors, a syringe with a blunt 18g needle, tube of glue, a silicone sleeve, leur lock bung and clamps. If glue is used in the repair of the catheter this has to be allowed to dry thoroughly before the catheter can be used again

Patient Education

1. Before discharge, patients and their carers should be taught how to safely manage the CVAD and be provided with written guidance to support this

2. Patients and their carers need to be aware of the signs and symptoms of infection. An awareness of potential complications and how to seek advice should also be established

References
National Health Service (2010). Guidelines for the Care and Maintenance of Central Venous Access Devices. Sutton and Merton NHS Trust: England.

Health Service Executive (2010). Guidelines for the Care and Maintenance of Long Term Central Venous Access Devices (CVAD's) in University Hospital Waterford excluding Dialysis Lines. UHW: Waterford.

University Hospital Waterford (2018). Guidelines for the Care and Maintenance of Long Term Central Venous Access Devices (CVAD's): UHW. Waterford.

60. Tunnelled Implanted Port-a-Cath Central Venous Access Devices (CVAD)-Blood Sampling

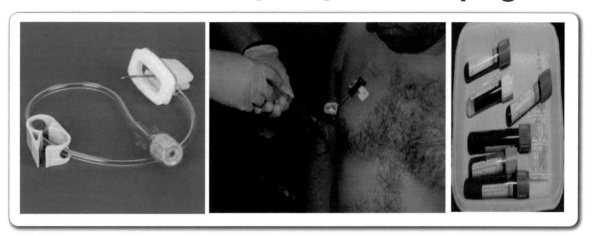

Equipment

- Dressing trolley (disinfected using large 70% alcohol wipe)

- Sterile dressing pack

- Sterile impervious sheet if not included in the dressing pack

- Antiseptic solution for skin disinfection (example Normasol)

- Port-a-Cath Gripper needle with extension set (appropriate guage)

- Individually wrapped needle free connector(s)

- Sterile gloves

- Required blood specimen bottles

- 10ml sterile leur lock syringe or 20ml leur lock syringe (if required) for blood sample or appropriate sterile vacutainer system compatible with gripper extension set

- 10ml sterile leur lock syringes and sterile needles x 3

- 10mls 0.9% sodium chloride for injection

- 4mls heparin sodium 100 iu/ml IV flush solution

- Sharps container

With each procedure adhere to standard precautions and use appropriate PPE e.g. gloves, goggles, apron as required

Check all equipment/preparations: do not use if packaging is contaminated or damaged or if expiry date is exceeded

Procedure

1. Identify the patient. Check patient's name, date of birth and hospital number against the patient's identification band if an in-patient. As an outpatient ascertain the patient's identity by verifying the name, date of birth and address

2. Provide the patient with privacy. Explain the procedure to the patient and give him/her the opportunity to voice concerns, preferences or ask questions

3. Where possible informed verbal consent must be obtained before beginning the Procedure

4. Check if the patient has any known allergies to skin preparations or adhesive material

5. Decontaminate hands according to correct hand hygiene techniques

6. Visually inspect entry/port site for signs of infection e.g. exudates /redness and /or tracking

7. Discuss observations with patient and check if they are experiencing any symptoms such as pain, swelling or tenderness at entry/port site

8. Locate the port and identify the septum

9. Open dressing pack taking care not to touch the inside of the sterile field, and open all of the sterile equipment aseptically onto the sterile field

10. Check contents, volume and expiry dates of the 0.9% sodium chloride and heparin solutions

11. Decontaminate hands and wrists and put on sterile gloves

12. Aseptically draw up the 0.9% sodium chloride and heparinised solutions from the vials. Remove needle and dispose directly into sharps container. Place syringes in sterile dish of dressing pack

13. Remove injection cap from the Port-a-Cath gripper needle and tubing before priming line with approximately 0.5ml of the 0.9% sodium chloride solution

14. Decontaminate the skin over the port with a single patient use application of antiseptic solution for skin disinfection (example Normasol)

15. Holding the gripper needle in the dominant hand stabilize the port between two fingers or thumb and finger of non-dominant hand

16. Inform the patient that you are about to insert the gripper needle

17. Insert the gripper needle at a 90 degree angle through the skin and port silicone septum until the Port-a-Cath needle is heard hitting the back of the titanium reservoir. This titanium reservoir cannot be perforated

18. Place the sterile impervious sheet under the gripper needle and extension tubing

19. Attach 10ml sterile leur lock syringe and withdraw back to check for blood return

20. Should no blood return refer to section on complications of CVAD's re partial or complete catheter occlusion

21. Once blood return is confirmed draw back 5-10 mls of blood and discard (in appropriate blood waste container)

Please note for coagulation studies up to 20mls of blood should be discarded or coagulation screen obtained as the last sample. If coagulation results appear to have been affected by heparin i.e. elevated, then the specimen should be repeated peripherally

22. Attach another 10ml or 20ml (if required) sterile leur lock syringe and draw back blood sample. Remove syringe and attach sterile needle

23. Inoculate blood carefully into the blood specimen bottle(s)

24. Remove needle and dispose directly into sharps container

25. Alternatively blood samples bottles can be filled directly using a compatible vacutainer system. Discard first 5-10 ml sample of blood or amounts as indicated above

26. Once blood sampling is complete the Port-a- Cath must be flushed

27. Using aseptic techniques flush the Port-a-Cath with 10mls of 0.9% sodium chloride using a push pause flow to maintain positive pressure

28. Flush with 4mls of heparin sodium 100 iu/ml IV flush solution as prescribed e.g. Heprinse, (using a push pause flow) clamping the line as the last ½ml is infusing to ensure positive pressure is maintained thus preventing backflow and clotting of blood

29. To remove the gripper needle immobilise the port between two fingers or thumb and finger of non-dominant hand. Remove needle with the dominant hand and dispose directly into sharps container

30. Apply pressure to the site with dry sterile gauze if ooze present after removing the needle. When ooze stopped discard used gauze in appropriate health care risk bag. Apply a small dressing to site if required

31. Dispose of all equipment appropriately, remove gloves and decontaminate hands.

32. Reconfirm patient details and label the blood sample bottles. Place samples in appropriate packaging/ lab transport receptacles and arrange transport of same

33. Ensure patient is comfortable

34. Document procedure fully in patient notes including date, time, any complications noted and signature of the Nurse carrying out the procedure

References

National Health Service (2010). Guidelines for the Care and Maintenance of Central Venous Access Devices. Sutton and Merton NHS Trust: England.

Health Service Executive (2010). Guidelines for the Care and Maintenance of Long Term Central Venous Access Devices (CVAD's) in University Hospital Waterford excluding Dialysis Lines. UHW: Waterford.

University Hospital Waterford (2018). Guidelines for the Care and Maintenance of Long Term Central Venous Access Devices (CVAD's). UHW: Waterford.

61. Tunnelled Central Venous Access Devices (CVAD) Hickman Catheters and PICC Lines Blood Sampling

Hickman Catheters

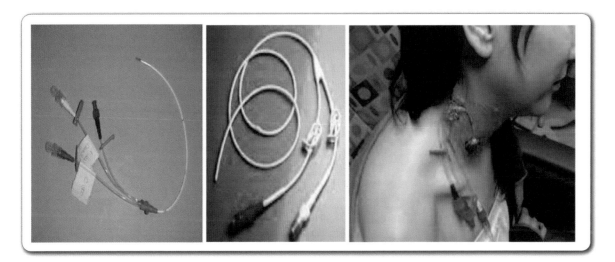

PICC Lines

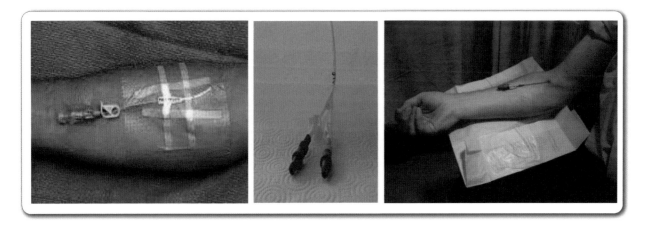

Equipment

- Dressing trolleyDressing trolley (disinfected using large 70% alcohol wipe)
- Sterile dressing pack
- Sterile impervious sheet if not included in the dressing pack
- Sterile gloves
- Individually wrapped large 2% chlorhexidine gluconate in isopropyl alcohol 70% wipes
- Individually wrapped small 70% isopropyl alcohol swabs if taking blood cultures

- 10ml sterile leur lock syringe or 20ml leur lock syringe (if required) for blood sample or appropriate sterile vacutainer system compatible with CVAD

- 10mls 0.9% sodium chloride for injection for each lumen of CVAD

- Heparin sodium 50iu/ml or 100iu/ml IV flush solution depending on type of CVAD lumen and individual patients prescription

  - **Hickman Catheter:** usually: 5mls of Heparin sodium 10iu/ml IV flush solution for each Hickman lumen clamping the catheter as the last ½ml is infusing to ensure that positive pressure is maintained, thus preventing backflow and clotting of blood. Always refer to patient's individual prescription and follow manufacturer's instructions

  - **PICC Line- usually:** 4mls of heparin sodium 100iu/ml IV flush solution clamping the catheter as the last ½ml is infusing for the same reasons as above. Always refer to patient's individual prescription and follow manufacturer's instructions

- Blood specimen bottles

- Sharps container

- With each procedure adhere to standard precautions and use appropriate PPE e.g. gloves, goggles, apron as required

Check all equipment/preparations

Do not use if packaging is contaminated or damaged or if expiry date is exceeded

Procedure

1. Identify the patient. Check patient's name, date of birth and hospital number against the patient's identification band if an in-patient. As an outpatient ascertain the patient's identity by verifying the name, date of birth and address

2. Provide the patient with privacy. Explain the procedure to the patient and give him/her the opportunity to voice concerns, preferences or ask questions

3. Where possible informed verbal consent must be obtained before beginning the procedure

4. Check if the patient has any known allergies to skin preparations or adhesive material

5. Check contents, volume and expiry dates of the 0.9% sodium chloride and heparin solutions

6. Decontaminate hands according to correct hand hygiene techniques

7. Open dressing pack taking care not to touch the inside of the sterile field, and open all of the sterile equipment aseptically onto the sterile field

8. Aseptically draw up the 0.9% sodium chloride and heparinised solutions from the vials. Remove needle and dispose directly into sharps container. Place syringes in sterile dish of dressing pack

9. Visually inspect CVAD entry/port site for signs of infection e.g. exudates /redness and /or tracking

10. Discuss observations with patient and check if they are experiencing any symptoms such as pain, swelling or tenderness at entry/port site

11. With a Hickman line ensure the dacron cuff is not visible at exit site. If it is and an infusion is in progress: turn off the infusion and clamp the catheter lumen. Decontaminate hands and wrists by applying an alcohol based hand-rub for 15 seconds e.g. Spirigel on clean hands. Put on sterile gloves, cover site with a sterile dressing and inform the medical team

Otherwise

12. If IV fluids infusing ensure that the line(s) is clamped for a maximum of 5 minutes before sampling occurs to avoid dilution of sample. Discard IV fluids once they are disconnected

13. Decontaminate hands and wrists using an alcohol based hand-rub e.g. Spirigel and put on sterile gloves

14. Place the sterile impervious sheet under the catheter line and needle free connector

15. Clean needle free connector using an individually wrapped large 2% chlorhexidine gluconate in 70% isopropyl alcohol wipe. Apply the wipe firmly and rotate five times over the silicone surface and associated rim of the device and allow the solution to air dry

16. Attach 10ml sterile leur lock syringe to needle free connector

17. Once blood return is confirmed draw back 5-10mls of blood and discard (in appropriate blood waste container). Should no blood return refer to section on complications of CVAD's re partial or complete catheter occlusion

Please note for coagulation studies up to 20mls of blood should be discarded or coagulation screen obtained as last sample. If coagulation results appear to have been affected by heparin i.e. elevated, then the specimen should be repeated peripherally

18. Attach another 10ml or 20ml (if required) sterile leur lock syringe and draw back blood sample. Remove syringe and attach sterile needle

19. Inoculate blood carefully into the blood specimen bottle(s). Immediately after filling the sample, remove needle and dispose directly into sharps container

20. Alternatively blood samples bottles can be filled directly using a CVAD compatible sterile vacutainer system. Discard first sample(s) or amounts as indicated above

21. Once blood sampling is complete the CVAD port(s) must be flushed

22. Using aseptic techniques flush line with 10mls of 0.9% sodium chloride followed by the appropriate heparin sodium IV flush as prescribed using a push pause technique (to maintain positive pressure) as per CVAD flushing guidelines

23. Dispose of all equipment appropriately, remove gloves and clean hands according to correct hand hygiene techniques

24. Reconfirm patient details and label the sample bottles. Place samples in appropriate packaging/ lab transport receptacles and arrange for transport of same

25. Ensure patient is comfortable

26. Document procedure fully in patient notes including date, time, any complications noted and signature of the Nurse carrying out the procedure

References

National Health Service (2010). Guidelines for the Care and Maintenance of Central Venous Access Devices. Sutton and Merton NHS Trust: England.

Health Service Executive (2010). Guidelines for the Care and Maintenance of Long Term Central Venous Access Devices (CVAD's) in University Hospital Waterford excluding Dialysis Lines. UHW: Waterford.

University Hospital Waterford (2018). Guidelines for the Care and Maintenance of Long Term Central Venous Access Devices (CVAD's). UHW: Waterford

62. Flushing Port-a-Cath Central Venous Access Devices (CVAD) Guidelines

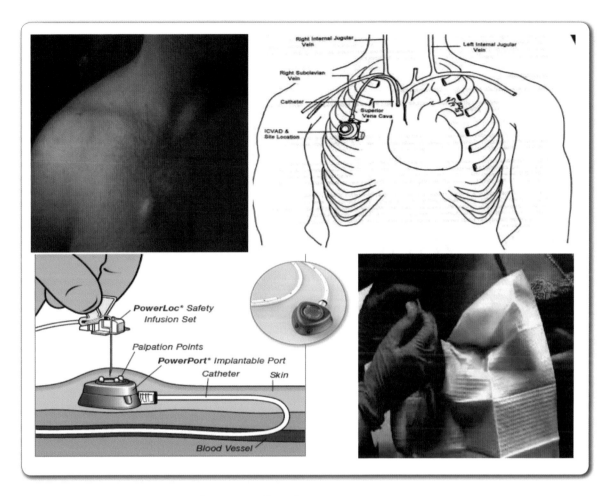

Tunnelled Implanted Ports (Port-a-Cath)

The Port-a-Cath tunnelled implantable port differs from other CVAD's because it has no external parts. The port sits under the patient's skin on the chest wall, lower rib cage or antecubital area. It is made up of a portal body and attached to a silicon catheter which sits in the lower third of the superior vena cava. It has a self-sealing septum which is accessed through intact skin and it can be used for long term vascular access (over 30 days).These devices have the lowest rates of catheter related blood stream infections.

The flushing of Port-a-Cath lines is carried out to help prevent vascular thrombosis, microbial adherence and Catheter related blood stream infection

Equipment

- Dressing trolley (disinfected using large 70% alcohol wipe)
- Sterile dressing pack
- Sterile impervious sheet if not included in the dressing pack
- Antiseptic solution for skin disinfection (example Normasol)
- Port-a-Cath Gripper needle with extension set (appropriate guage)
- Individually wrapped needle free connector(s)
- Sterile gloves
- 10ml sterile leur lock syringes and sterile needles x 3
- 10mls 0.9% sodium chloride for injection
- 4mls heparin sodium 100 iu/ml IV flush solution e.g. Heprinse
- Sharps container

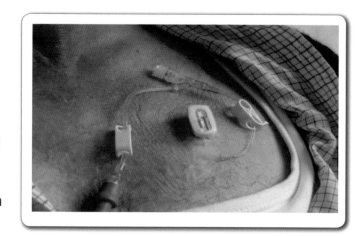

Procedure

1. Identify the patient. Check patient's name, date of birth and hospital number against the patient's identification band if an in-patient. As an outpatient ascertain the patient's identity by verifying the name, date of birth and address

2. Provide the patient with privacy. Explain the procedure to the patient and give him/her the opportunity to voice concerns, preferences or ask questions

3. Where possible informed verbal consent must be obtained before beginning the procedure

4. Check if the patient has any known allergies to skin preparations or adhesive material

5. Decontaminate hands according to correct hand hygiene techniques

6. Visually inspect entry/port site for signs of infection e.g. exudates /redness and /or tracking

7. Discuss observations with patient and check if they are experiencing any symptoms such as pain, swelling or tenderness at entry/port site

8. Locate the port and identify the septum

9. Open dressing pack taking care not to touch the inside of the sterile field, and open all of the sterile equipment aseptically onto the sterile field

10. Check contents, volume and expiry dates of the 0.9% sodium chloride and heparin solutions

11. Decontaminate hands and wrists as above and put on sterile gloves

12. Aseptically draw up the 0.9% sodium chloride and heparinised solutions from the vials. Remove needle and dispose directly into sharps container. Place syringes in sterile dish of dressing pack

13. Remove injection cap from the Port-a-Cath gripper needle and tubing before priming line with approximately 0.5ml of the 0.9% sodium chloride solution

14. Decontaminate the skin over the port with a single patient use application of antiseptic solution for skin disinfection (example Normasol)

15. Holding the gripper needle in the dominant hand stabilize the port between two fingers or thumb and finger of non-dominant hand

16. Inform the patient that you are about to insert the gripper needle

17. Insert the gripper needle at a 90 degree angle through the skin and port silicone septum until the Port-a-Cath needle is heard hitting the back of the titanium reservoir. This titanium reservoir cannot be perforated

18. Place the sterile impervious sheet under the gripper needle and extension tubing

19. Attach 10ml sterile leur lock syringe and withdraw back to check for blood return

20. Should no blood return refer to section on complications of CVAD's re partial or complete catheter occlusion

21. Once blood return is present commence flushing the port

22. Flush the Port-a-Cath with 10mls of 0.9% sodium chloride using a push pause flow to maintain positive pressure.

23. Flush with 4mls of heparin sodium 100 iu/ml IV flush solution as prescribed e.g. Heprinse, (using a push pause flow) clamping the line as the last ½ml is infusing to ensure positive pressure is maintained thus preventing backflow and clotting of blood

24. To remove the gripper needle immobilise the port between two fingers or thumb and finger of non-dominant hand. Remove needle with the dominant hand and dispose directly into sharps container

25. Apply pressure to the site with dry sterile gauze if ooze present after removing the needle. When ooze stopped discard used gauze in appropriate health care risk bag. Apply a small dressing to site if required

26. Dispose of all equipment appropriately, remove gloves and decontaminate hands according to correct hand hygiene techniques

27. Ensure patient is comfortable

28. Document procedure fully in patient notes including date, time, any complications noted and signature of the Nurse carrying out the procedure

References

National Health Service (2010). Guidelines for the Care and Maintenance of Central Venous Access Devices. Sutton and Merton NHS Trust: England.

Health Service Executive (2010). Guidelines for the Care and Maintenance of Long Term Central Venous Access Devices (CVAD's) in University Hospital Waterford excluding Dialysis Lines. UHW: Waterford.

University Hospital Waterford (2018). Guidelines for the Care and Maintenance of Long Term Central Venous Access Devices (CVAD's). UHW: Waterford.

Note: A gripper needle can be left in situ for up to seven days when in regular use
When not in regular use tunnelled implanted ports (Port-a-Cath's) should be flushed every four weeks

63. Female Catheterisation Guidelines

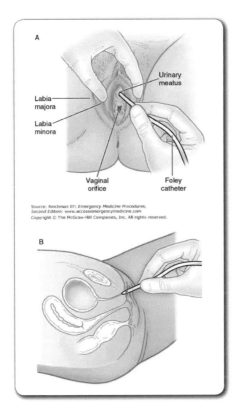

A

Urinary meatus

Labia majora

Labia minora

Vaginal orifice

Foley catheter

Source: Reichman EF: *Emergency Medicine Procedures, Second Edition*: www.accessemergencymedicine.com
Copyright © The McGraw-Hill Companies, Inc. All rights reserved.

B

Equipment

- Trolley
- Sterile gloves x2 pairs
- Plastic apron
- Cleansing solution e.g. Saline
- Catheterisation pack- Sterile
- Foley catheter (appropriate size and material)
- Anaesthetic / lubricating gel with nozzle (single use/ sterile)
- Syringe (usually 10 cc) and needle if applicable
- Sterile water (usually 10 cc)
- Universal container/ receiver
- Drainage bag and tubing / Securing straps and or catheter stand

Procedure

1. Explain procedure to the patient and gain informed consent
2. Decontaminate hands using correct hand hygiene techniques
3. Prepare trolley, placing all equipment required on the bottom shelf
4. Ensure patient privacy
5. Assist patient into supine position with knees bent, hips flexed and feet resting about 60 cm apart
6. Decontaminate hands using correct hand hygiene techniques
7. Put on apron and gloves and prepare the sterile field

8. Using aseptic technique open sterile catheter pack and appropriately sized Foley catheter and place on the sterile field

9. Use sterile drapes to cover patient and create sterile field

10. Using gauze swabs separate the labia minora so that the urethral meatus is seen

11. Clean around the urethral orifice with 0.9% NACL using single downward strokes

12. Place a small amount of the lubricating jelly/anaesthetic gel onto the tip of the catheter

13. Place the catheter in the sterile receiver between the patients legs

14. Introduce the tip of the catheter into the urethral orifice in an upward and backward direction. Advance the catheter until 5-6 cm has been inserted

15. If patient complains of any pain or discomfort stop and seek medical advice

16. If there is no urine present, remove the catheter gently and start procedure again. If urine is present, advance the catheter 6-8 cm

17. Gently inflate the balloon with required amount of sterile water (usually 10cc) or appropriate solution according to the manufacturer's instructions

18. Observe the patient for any signs of discomfort

19. Inflation should be pain free. If pain occurs deflate the balloon and insert the catheter slightly further into the urethra

20. Withdraw the catheter gently until the balloon is positioned against the bladder wall

21. Attach catheter to the drainage bag or catheter valve. Ensure patient is comfortable

22. Secure the catheter and position drainage bag below the level of the bladder

23. Support the catheter if required by taping the catheter to the patients leg or by using a specially designed support

24. Evaluate catheter function and record amount, colour, odour, and quality of urine

25. If required take a urine sample for lab analysis

26. Remove gloves and dispose of all equipment appropriately in the correct waste

27. Decontaminate hands according to correct hand hygiene techniques

28. Document the procedure including;

- Date and time of insertion
- Catheter type, length, balloon size and gauge
- Batch number
- Cleaning solution used
- Type of anaesthetic lubricant gel
- Amount of sterile water used to inflate the balloon
- Name and signature of nurse carrying out the procedure
- Any problems encountered during insertion
- Urinary output on insertion
- Date for removal/ change

References
Health Service Executive (2017). Clinical Competence in Female Catheterisation. Continence Promotion Unit. Dr Steven's Hospital, HSE: Dublin

64. Male Catheterisation Guidelines

Indications

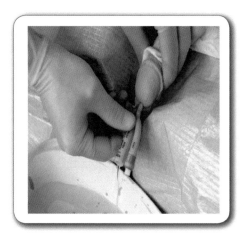

- Urinary retention
- To monitor urinary output (CCF/ Shock)
- To bypass an obstruction
- To ensure complete bladder emptying
- To allow bladder function tests (urodynamics)
- Bladder irrigation
- Measurement of residual urine
- Pre and post operatively
- Changing long term indwelling catheter
- To introduce cytotoxic drugs
- Intractable incontinence when no other means suitable

Contraindications

1. Known history of obstruction/ trauma requiring medical assistance
2. Stent or artificial urinary sphincter in situ
3. History of trauma (pelvic or abdominal trauma; urethral stricture; carcinoma of the lower urinary tract; abdominal penile discharge; congenital abnormalities example hydrospadies/epispadies; gross haematuria)
4. Patients< 48 hrs post TURP
5. Priapism (due to sickle cell or other disease)
6. Personal or physiological rejection of catheter

Prior to male catheterisation observe;

- Hygiene of the meatus and foreskin
- Meatal erosion, bleeding, sores or inflammation
- Paraphimosis, balanitis
- Scrotal, hydrocele, orchitis or swellings
- Conditions of the skin around the groin and scrotal area

Equipment

- Trolley
- Sterile gloves x2 pairs
- Plastic apron
- Cleansing solution e.g. Saline
- Catheterisation pack- sterile
- Foley catheter (appropriate size and material)
- Anaesthetic / lubricating gel with nozzle (single use/sterile)
- Syringe (usually 10 cc) and needle if applicable
- Sterile water (usually 10 cc) Universal container/ receiver
- Drainage bag and tubing / Securing straps and or catheter stand

Procedure

1. Explain procedure to the patient and gain informed consent
2. Prepare equipment.
3. Ensure patient privacy
4. Assist patient into supine position with legs extended
5. Decontaminate hands according to correct hand hygiene techniques
6. Put on apron and gloves and prepare sterile field
7. Open catheterisation pack
8. Repeat hand washing and put on sterile gloves
9. Use sterile drapes to cover patient and create sterile field.
10. Retract the foreskin and clean the glans penis with saline
11. Apply a small amount of the anaesthetic gel to tip of penis and then insert the nozzle of the lubricating anaesthetic gel into the urethra
12. Hold the glans firmly for a few minutes (5 mins) to allow the gel to work and prevent leaking
13. Wipe the underside of the penile shaft with dry gauze in a downward motion to move gel towards the prostatic urethra

14. Repeat hand washing and apply new sterile gloves

15. Place the receiver containing the catheter on a sterile towel under the penis

16. Open the catheter

17. Hold the penis firmly in the non-dominant hand rising it (perpendicular to patient's body) until it is almost fully extended

18. Hold the catheter in the dominant hand and pass it into the urethral meatus

19. Gently insert through the urethra into the bladder

20. If patient complains of any pain or discomfort stop and seek medical advice

21. If resistance is felt at the external sphincter ask the patient to cough or strain gently as if they were trying to pass urine

22. Then try to insert the catheter gently into the bladder

23. If resistance continues or the patient complains of discomfort or pain or bleeding occurs stop the procedure and seek medical advice

24. Insert catheter 15-25 cm or until urine begins to flow

25. Insert catheter almost to its bifurcation before inflating balloon to make sure the catheter has cleared the prostatic bed and is in the bladder

26. Gently inflate the balloon with required amount of sterile water (usually 10cc) or appropriate solution according to the manufacturer's instructions

27. Observe the patient for any signs of discomfort

28. Inflation should be pain free. If pain occurs deflate the balloon and insert the catheter slightly further into the urethra

29. Withdraw the catheter gently until the balloon is positioned against the bladder wall

30. Attach catheter to the drainage bag or catheter valve

31. Reposition the foreskin

32. Ensure the patient is comfortable and the area is dry

33. Secure the catheter and position drainage bag below the level of the bladder

34. Evaluate catheter function and amount, colour, odour, and quality of urine

35. Remove gloves and dispose of equipment appropriately

36. Decontaminate hands according to correct hand hygiene techniques

37. Document the procedure including;

- Date and time of insertion
- Catheter type, length, balloon size and gauge
- Batch number
- Cleaning solution used
- Type of anaesthetic lubricant gel
- Amount of sterile water used to inflate the balloon
- Name and signature of nurse carrying out the procedure
- Any problems encountered during insertion
- Urinary output on insertion
- Date for removal/ change

References
Health Service Executive (2017). Clinical Competence in Male Adult Urethral Catheterisation. Continence Promotion Unit. Dr Steeven's Hospital. HSE: Dublin

65. Suprapubic Re-Catheterisation Guidelines

The first change of a suprapubic catheter occurs in hospital

Equipment

- Catheterisation pack
- Non sterile gloves
- Two pairs of sterile gloves
- Plastic disposable apron
- Catheters of appropriate size (100% Silicone / Hydrogel latex long term). 100% silicone catheters are more prone to cuffing
- Sterile lubricating gel
- Saline or antiseptic solution for abdominal cleaning
- 10mls of sterile water for balloon inflation (some catheters have pre-filled 10ml syringe included) 10ml syringe x 2
- Sterile drainage bag
- Universal specimen container (if required)

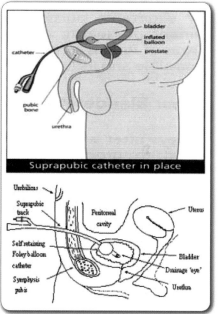

Procedure

1. Explain procedure to the patient and gain informed consent
2. Prepare equipment.
3. Ensure patient privacy
4. Assist patient into supine position
5. Decontaminate hands according to correct hand hygiene techniques
6. Urine bag should be clamped for approximately 5 minutes prior to removal of catheter
7. Apply non-sterile gloves. Deflate balloon slowly with 10 ml syringe; wait 3 minutes before removing
8. Remove non-sterile gloves. Wash and dry hands
9. Prepare sterile field
10. Open catheter pack and required equipment onto sterile field

11. Apply sterile gloves and lubricate new catheter tip with sterile lubricating gel

12. Apply sterile protective sheet/ drape

13. Clean the area at site of catheter with normal saline

14. Having deflated the balloon, remove indwelling catheter taking note of angle and length of catheter

15. Leave catheter aside to check for encrustation

16. Remove gloves and wash hands. Apply sterile gloves

17. Apply sterile protective sheet over supra-pubic site

18. Immediately insert the new catheter into the supra-pubic opening at the same angle and length as the previous catheter

19. Check that urine is draining before inflating the balloon with 10mls of sterile water

20. Attach sterile bag

21. Remove gloves and decontaminate hands according to correct hand hygiene techniques

22. Make the patient comfortable. Advise patient re catheter care, change of catheter date, potential complications and what to do in an emergency

23. Document the procedure. Attach batch sticker from packaging to patients chart if applicable and or record type, size and batch number of catheter on electronic notes

24. Dispose of clinical waste appropriately

References
Health Service Executive (2017). Suprapubic Re-catheterisation. Clinical Competence in Catheterisation. Continence Promotion Unit. Dr Steeven's Hospital, HSE: Dublin

66. Indwelling Catheter Irrigation Guidelines

Indicated to reduce or dissolve encrustation or crystallisation in the catheter or bladder. For use once weekly to maximum twice daily depending on the severity of the case or as prescribed by the Doctor

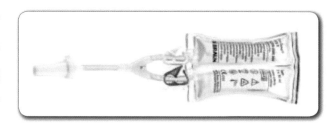

Equipment

- Prescription for irrigation solution
- Irrigation solution (eg SubyG) (correct strength) as charted on the prescription Catheter pack
- Absorbent sheet Clamp
- Cleaning solution eg Normasol New catheter bag (leg bag)
- Container of warm water for warming the catheter flushing solution
- Gloves
- Apron
- Clinical waste disposal bag

Procedure

1. Explain the procedure to the patient and gain informed consent
2. Ensure the patient is in a comfortable position
3. Warm the irrigation solution to body temperature by immersing in warm water
4. Expose the catheter and observe for any signs of discharge
5. Decontaminate hands using correct hand-washing technique and put on the gloves and apron
6. Open the catheter pack and using aseptic / clean techniques cleanse the indwelling catheter with an appropriate cleaning solution eg. Normasol
7. Clamp the indwelling catheter and place the absorbent sheet under the catheter junction
8. Close the clamp and remove the cover of the catheter irrigation solution without touching the tip
9. Disconnect the drainage bag and insert the catheter irrigation solution into the catheter

10. Follow the manufacturer's instructions for the administration of the irrigation solution, volume to be administered, and time for retention of the solution

11. Slide the clamp open on the catheter irrigation solution, raise the bag slightly above the level of the bladder and allow the required amount of the solution to flow into the bladder. Gentle pressure may be needed taking care initially to start the flow (rapid instillation of fluid may be uncomfortable for the patient)

12. If the fluid is not going into the bladder don't force it; instead squeeze the catheter tubing gently to break down the sediment and try again

13. Observe during administration for bypassing around the catheter, bleeding or bladder spasm resulting in inability to retain the solution

14. Stop administration if the patient becomes distressed or finds the procedure painful or uncomfortable

15. Retain the fluid for the period of time indicated, close the clamp and place the bag on the bed. Ensure the patient is comfortable for the required time

16. When the catheter flushing solution is to be removed, ensure the bag / chamber is below the level of the bladder (for gravity to facilitate drainage), open the clamp and allow the solution to drain back into the chamber/bag

17. Some irrigation fluid administration sets have two irrigation chambers/ bags for infusion

18. When all the solution has drained back out of the bladder, close the clamp (to prevent spillage of the solution) disconnect the solution container and connect a new catheter leg drainage bag

19. If the solution does not drain out, reposition the patient

20. Note the amount of fluid returned

21. Make the patient comfortable

22. Remove and dispose of equipment correctly in appropriate waste bags

23. Decontaminate hands using correct hand-washing technique

24. Document the procedure and report any complications if relevant

References
Cheshire Ireland (2013). Standard Procedure for the Irrigating (flushing) of an Indwelling Catheter, Document Number: CLSP 29, Version Number: 2, Version Date: 31/05/2013. Cheshire Ireland

67. Nephrostomy Tube: Dressing and Bag Change

Equipment

- 0.9% NACL
- Drainage bag and leg straps
- Non-sterile gloves
- Dressing pack with gauze
- Disposable plastic apron
- Drain fixation dressing
- Bactericidal alcohol hand-rub
- Clamp (blunt disposable)
- Alcohol (chlorhexidine) wipe
- Adhesive remover
- Micropore tape

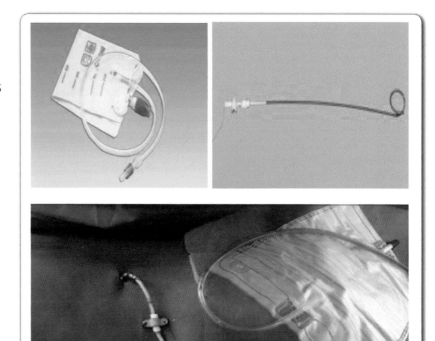

Procedure

1. Explain and discuss the procedure with the patient and gain informed consent
2. Position the patient comfortably and provide privacy
3. Decontaminate hands using correct hand hygiene techniques
4. Put on a disposable plastic apron and gloves
5. Prepare the dressing trolley placing all equipment required on the bottom shelf
6. Assist the patient onto the edge of the bed/couch sitting in an upright position with their back exposed
7. Keeping the drain secure with one hand, carefully remove existing drain fixation dressing and inspect the incisions site. Check sutures remain intact
8. Pour a small amount of adhesive remover onto a gauze square. Keeping the drain secure with one hand, use the adhesive remover to remove any dressing residue from the drain tubing
9. Clean hands according to correct hand hygiene techniques

10. Put on sterile gloves

11. Clean the drain site with 0.9% NACL, working from the drain outwards. Gently remove any encrustation. Allow the site to dry

12. When the site is dry, apply a sterile drain fixation dressing according to manufacturer's guidelines. Window frame the edges of the dressing to prevent it rucking by applying surgical tape around the edges of the dressing

13. Decontaminate hands according to correct hand hygiene techniques

14. Gently clamp nephrostomy tube using blunt disposable clamp (if available)

15. Disconnect the drainage bag, and connector if attached, from the nephrostomy tube

16. Clean connector hub with alcohol-impregnated chlorhexidine wipe

17. Apply new sterile drainage bag, and connector if required, to the nephrostomy tube, being careful not to touch the hubs and unclamp the drain. Urine should begin to flow

18. Apply leg or waist strap according to patient preference to secure the bag to the patient. Ensure the tube is not taut or pulling at the exit site

19. Dispose of waste correctly in the clinical waste bag

20. Decontaminate hands according to correct hand hygiene techniques

21. Ensure the patient is comfortable post procedure

22. Record the procedure in the patients records, including

   - Date and time of procedure

   - Procedure/s performed

   - Dressing and bag type used

   - Condition of the skin

   - Any problems or concerns during the procedure

   - Any swabs/samples taken during the procedure

   - Referrals made

   - Review date for next dressing/bag change

References
Health Service Executive (2017). Clinical Competence in Catheterisation. Continence Promotion Unit. Dr Steven's Hospital. HSE: Dublin.

68. PEG Tube Insertion Guidelines Inserting Corflo Replacement Gastrostomy Tubes

Important

If the original PEG tube falls out in the first 3 weeks of placement, cover stoma site and arrange for transfer to Hospital for endoscopy. Do not attempt to put a catheter or a replacement PEG in the stoma site, as the site is immature. The patient needs to be off anticoagulants for 7 days prior to endoscopy/ PEG tube re-insertion.

If the original PEG falls out between 4 and 6 weeks of placement, keep the stoma open (example with a Foley Catheter- see separate guidelines for emergency gastrostomy replacement with balloon tube) and transfer to hospital, as the tract is not formed and replacement tubes may be placed incorrectly. A new tube may have to be placed endoscopically.

Equipment

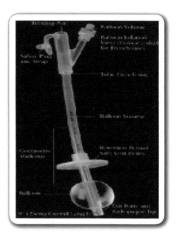

- Replacement Corflo Gastrostomy tube packs (various sizes)
- Sterile water
- Dressing pack
- 0.05% chlorahexidine solution
- 10ml syringe
- pH indicator strips
- 50 ml syringe (single use only)
- Clean disposable plastic apron
- Gloves
- Paper towel
- Gastrostomy tube / Balloon sizes
- 12F = 5cc
- 14F= 5cc
- 16F=5cc / 16F= 20cc (check pack instructions as some size 16's differ) 18F=5cc
- 20F= 20c

Procedure

1. Check date of insertion and size of original PEG tube in medical chart (Must be > 6 weeks for fistulisation)

2. Explain procedure and obtain consent from patient or carer

3. Decontaminate hands using correct hand hygiene techniques. Don disposable gloves, apron and other PPE as appropriate

4. Open a dressing pack and set up on a clinically clean trolley

5. Check expiration date and size of replacement gastrostomy tube

6. Open gastrostomy set and check that the balloon inflates prior to inflation and move the bolster up and down the tube

7. Coat tip of replacement tube with water soluble lubricated gel

8. Soak gauze in 0.05% chlorhexidine solution and clean area around stoma

9. Protect the patient with a paper towel

10. Deflate Replacement Gastrostomy Tube by removing all water from the balloon using a 10 ml syringe, making sure the balloon is fully deflated prior to removal of the tube

11. Remove the Replacement Gastrostomy Tube. Discard the tube in yellow bag. If gloved hands have become contaminated following removal of the Gastrostomy Tube, remove, decontaminate hands and don gloves

12. Using non touch aseptic technique, clean around site using 0.05% chlorhexidine

13. Insert the same size tube as the tube that has been removed. If this fails, try a smaller size tube

14. Insert tube into stoma, up to the end of the writing on the tube (past the 6cm mark on the tube)

15. Check balloon volume. Inflate tube with the correct volume of sterile water

16. Pull the replacement tube back so that balloon is resting inside stomach wall

17. Slide retention bolster to stoma/skin surface

18. Wipe off excess lubricating gel around the stoma site using gauze

19. Aspirate Replacement Gastrostomy Tube. Check tube placement with pH indicator strips. If pH is less than 5.5 can feed immediately. If pH higher than 5.5, wait for 30 minutes and retest. If the patient is on antacids or proton pump inhibitors, pH may be higher, wait for 30 minutes and re-test

20. Place side clamp on tube

21. Flush tube with 30mls of sterile water

If the patient experiences any pain on flushing of the Replacement Gastrostomy Tube post PEG replacement, STOP, do not put any medications or feed down the tube. Repeat steps 10-

20. An X-Ray is not required. However, if the patient continues to experience any pain arrange transfer to Hospital

22. Close feeding port

29. Dispose of waste into appropriate waste streams. Remove PPE and decontaminate hands according to correct hand hygiene techniques

23. Decontaminate reusable items of equipment

24. Document procedure in clinical notes

References

St Luke's Hospital (2011). Guidelines for Enteral Feeding, St Luke's Hospital, Kilkenny. Ireland.

St Luke's Hospital (2013). Policies and Procedures: Revised Guidelines for Enteral Feeding. Inserting Corflo Replacement Gastrostomy tubes, St Luke's Hospital. Kilkenny, Ireland.

69. Emergency Gastrostomy Replacement with Balloon Tube (Example Foley Catheter)

If an existing Gastrostomy (PEG) tube has fallen out, or been accidentally pulled out, the stoma will close quickly, often in the space of a few hours. It is important that a tube is reinserted as soon as possible to prevent the stoma closing.

Initial/First insertion PEG tubes must be replaced by the hospital

If the gastrostomy tube has been in place less than 6 weeks a mature track may not have formed and the risks of inadvertently placing the replacement tube in the peritoneal cavity are high. A mature track can take many weeks to form, especially in a malnourished patient.

If the original PEG tube falls out in the first weeks after the primary insertion/placement do not insert anything into the stoma. Re-admit the patient. Seek advice from the hospital, on-call radiologist or surgeon.

Note: A urinary catheter is just a temporary measure and not appropriate for long term use as a Gastrostomy tube. Once a urinary catheter has been inserted appropriate arrangements should be made for this to be changed to a Gastrostomy (PEG) tube as soon as possible

Equipment

- Dressing Trolley
- Sterile gloves
- Plastic apron
- Cleansing solution e.g. Saline/ Normasol
- Catheterisation pack- sterile
- Foley catheter (appropriate size)
- Anaesthetic / lubricating gel with nozzle (single use/sterile)
- Syringe (10 ml) and needle if applicable
- Sterile water (10 mls)
- 50 ml syringe (to check for gastric aspirate)
- pH indicator strips
- Clinical waste bag

Procedure

1. Check date of insertion and size of original PEG tube. (Must be in place longer than 6 weeks for fistulisation to occur)

   Note: all initial/ first time PEG tube replacements must be carried out at the hospital)

2. Explain the procedure to the patient and gain informed consent

3. Place the patient in a lying position or straight with the bed tilted head up

4. Decontaminate hands using correct technique and put on apron and gloves

5. Open the Catheter pack and Foley Catheter (correct size)

6. Clean the external gastrostomy site /stoma with appropriate cleansing solution example Saline/ Normasol

7. Lubricate the stoma track with local anaesthetic gel

8. Gently insert the Foley catheter tube through the stoma track **(Do not use any force)**. The track is often not perpendicular to the skin and if the tube will not pass easily into the stomach the direction of the track can be reassessed using a narrower (smaller) urinary catheter. **Do not force it in**. It should go easily into the track for 4-5cms or at least the length of the track as assessed by the removed Gastrostomy tube

9. If the stoma has started to close you may need to use a narrower Foley catheter tube to keep the stoma patent in the short term. If the track needs dilatation this should only be done by appropriately trained medical or surgical staff

10. Once the Foley catheter/ tube has been passed into the stomach it should rotate freely. The tube/ catheter should be advanced at least 2 to 3cms further in than the position of the displaced tube

11. Inflate the catheter balloon with water (usually 10mls) according to the instructions. Inflation should not cause pain

12. Gently pull the catheter tube back until there is resistance (when the internal balloon comes up against the stomach wall)

13. Secure the catheter in position with tape to the skin. Externally fixing the catheter tube prevents the internal balloon being pulled into the pylorus or duodenum. If this happens it can result in gastric secretions or feeds being vomited or leaking around the tube

14. Aspirate catheter tube for gastric fluids (to ensure tube is in the stomach) and check aspirate with pH indicator strips

15. Ensure the patient is comfortable post procedure

16. Dispose of all waste equipment appropriately in clinical waste bags

17. Decontaminate hands according to correct hand hygiene techniques

18. Document procedure and report any complications which may have occurred during the procedure

References

St Luke's Hospital (2011). Guidelines for Enteral Feeding, St Luke's Hospital, Kilkenny. Ireland.

St Luke's Hospital (2013). Policies and Procedures: Emergency Gastrostomy Replacement with Balloon Tube. St Luke's Hospital. Kilkenny, Ireland

70. Insertion of Replacement Corflo Cubby low profile Gastrostomy (PEG) Device (LPGD)

Equipment

- Corflo Cubby LPGD's in various sizes
- Corflo Cubby Stoma measuring device
- Water soluble lubricating jelly
- 10mls Sterile water
- Dressing pack
- 0.05% chlorhexidine solution
- 10ml syringe
- Clean disposable plastic apron
- Gloves (non-sterile)
- Paper towel

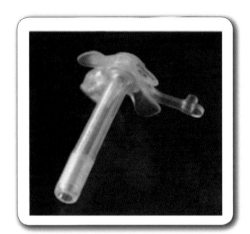

Procedure

1. Check date of insertion and size of original PEG tube in medical chart. (Must be > 6 weeks for fistulization)
2. Explain procedure and obtain consent from patient or carer
3. Decontaminate hands according to correct hand hygiene techniques
4. Don disposable gloves, apron and other PPE as appropriate
5. Deflate balloon in existing replacement gastrostomy tube or button by removing the water using 10 ml syringe
6. Clean area surrounding the stoma, using non touch aseptic technique with 0.05% chlorhexidine solution
7. Check balloon inflates on stoma measuring device
8. Lubricate the tip of the measuring device with water soluble lubricant
9. Gentle slide the tip of the measuring device through the stoma site into the stomach
10. Use the Luer lock syringe provided to inflate the balloon with 5mls Turn the stopcock 90 degrees to retain the air in the balloon

11. Place gentle traction on the measuring device until you feel resistance against the inside stomach wall

12. It is recommended to take two readings, one in the upright and one in the supine position. Take the average of the two readings for the desired length. Measurements are in 0.5 cm increments

13. Record the appropriate length. It is important to select the appropriate length for the abdominal wall thickness. If measurement is between sizes, choose the next larger size

14. **Warning: Under sizing the Corflo-Cubby may cause embedding with erosion into the gastric wall, tissue necrosis, infection, abscess, sepsis and associated sequelae**

15. Deflate the balloon and remove the measuring device. If gloved hands have become contaminated following removal of the tube, remove, decontaminate hands and don new gloves

16. Select the appropriate size Corflo Cubby. Check that the balloon inflates

17. Using a non-touch aseptic technique, clean around site using 0.05% chlorhexidine

18. Coat tip of replacement tube with water lubricated gel. Insert tube into stoma

19. Hold firmly in place and inflate balloon with the 5mls of sterile water

20. Close feeding port

21. Dispose of waste appropriately, remove PPE and decontaminate hands according to correct hand hygiene techniques

22. Document the procedure in the patients notes

23. Educate patient/carer on use of Corflo Cubby LPGD

24. An X-Ray is not required

References
St Luke's Hospital (2013). Policies and Procedures: Revised Guidelines for Enteral Feeding. Inserting Corflo Replacement Cubby Gastrostomy tubes.

Document Reference No: SLGH DTN 001 Revision No: 1 Approval Date: Nov 2013. St Luke's Hospital. Kilkenny, Ireland

71. Insertion of a Nasogastric (NG) Tube

Equipment

- Clean tray
- Receiver
- Nasogastric tube
- Drainage bag
- Tape
- Disposable gloves
- Apron
- Lubricating jelly
- Gauze squares
- 50 ml syringe

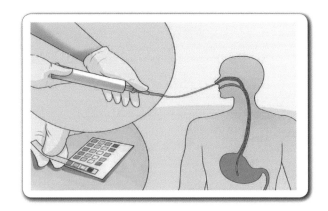

Procedure

1. Explain and discuss the procedure with the patient. Gain informed consent

2. Arrange a signal by which the patient can communicate with the nurse to stop the procedure, example by raising their hand

3. Assist the patient to sit in a semi-upright position. Place a pillow behind their head for support. The head should not be tilted backwards or forwards

4. To identify the length of tube that needs to be inserted, use a small piece of tape to mark the distance to which the tube is to be passed, by measuring the distance on the tube from the patients earlobe to the bridge of the nose, plus the distance from the earlobe to the xiphisternum

5. Decontaminate hands according to correct hand hygiene techniques and put on disposable gloves and apron

6. Check the nostrils are patent by asking the patient to sniff with one nostril closed. Repeat with the other nostril

7. Lubricate about 15-20 cm of the tube with a thin coat of lubricating jelly that has been placed on a gauze swab

8. To prevent spillage and reduce the risk of infection, ensure the receiver is placed beneath the end of the tube

9. Insert the proximal end of the tube into the clearer nostril and slide it backwards and inwards along the floor of the nose to the nasopharynx. If an obstruction is felt, withdraw the tube and try again in a slightly different direction or use the other nostril

10. As the tube passes down the nasopharynx, ask the patient to start swallowing. Offer sips of water

11. Advance the tube through the pharynx as the patient swallows until the tape marked tube reaches the point of entry into the nostril. If the patient shows signs of distress for example gasping or cyanosis, remove the tube immediately

12. Secure the tube to the nostril with adherent dressing tape or a hypoallergenic tape if required. Secure the tube to the cheek with an adhesive patch

13. Use the syringe to gently aspirate any stomach contents and then attach the tube to a drainage bag

14. If unsure of the tubes position, aspirate 0.5 – 1 ml of aspirate and test the pH using indicator strips. A pH of between 1 and 5.5 reflects the acidity of the stomach and is unlikely to be pulmonary aspirate

15. Ensure the patient is comfortable post procedure

16. Remove gloves and apron and dispose of all equipment safely

17. Decontaminate hands using correct hand hygiene techniques

18. Document the procedure in the patients notes, including NEX measurement and length of visible portion of the tube from tip of nose

Source: Dougherty, L. & Lister, S. (2015) The Royal Marsden Hospital Manual of Clinical Nursing Procedures. 9th Ed. Wiley Blackwell Pub: Chichester

72.Removal of a Nasogastric (NG) Tube

Equipment

- Clean gloves and apron
- Clinical/ contaminated waste disposal bag
- Bowl of warm water and wipes

Procedure

1. Explain and discuss the procedure with the patient. Gain informed consent
2. Assist the patient to sit in a semi-upright position. Place a pillow behind their head for support.
3. Decontaminate hands according to correct hand hygiene techniques and assemble the equipment required
4. Apply apron and gloves
5. Remove any tape securing the nasogastric tube to the face and nose
6. Using a steady and constant motion, gently pull the tube until it has been completely removed
7. Place the used nasogastric tube directly into the contaminated clinical waste bag
8. Using warm water and wipes, clean the nose and face to remove any traces of tape
9. Assist the patient to find a comfortable position
10. Remove gloves and apron and dispose of all equipment safely
11. Decontaminate hands using correct hand hygiene techniques
12. Document the procedure in the patients records

73. Stoma Bag Change Guidelines

Equipment

- Clean tray or trolley
- Tissues
- Wipes
- Adhesive remover
- New stoma bag and seals
- Measuring device/template
- Scissors
- Clinical waste disposal bags
- Bowl of warm water
- Soap
- Gloves and apron
- Jug (if drainable bag used)

Procedure

1. Explain and discuss the procedure with the patient and gain informed consent

2. Ensure that the patient is in a suitable and comfortable position where they will be able to see the procedure (if teaching the patient). A mirror may be used to aid visualisation

3. Set up the trolley/ tray with the required equipment

4. Decontaminate hands according to correct hand hygiene techniques

5. Use a protective pad /sheet to protect the patients clothing from drips if the effluent is fluid and apply gloves and apron

6. If the bag is a drainable type, empty the contents into a jug before removing the bag

7. Remove the appliance slowly. Peel the adhesive off the skin with one hand while exerting gentle pressure on the skin with the other

8. Fold appliance in two to ensure no spillage and place in disposal bag

9. Remove excess faeces or mucus from the stoma with a damp tissue

10. Examine the skin and stoma for soreness, bleeding or ulceration. If the skin is unblemished and the stoma is a healthy red colour proceed

11. Wash the skin and stoma gently until clean

12. Dry the skin and stoma gently but thoroughly

13. Measure the stoma and cut appliance, leaving 3mm clearance

14. Apply the new stoma bag, ensuring a good seal with the skin. The appliance should provide skin protection when attached properly and the aperture is cut just a little larger than the stoma so that effluent cannot cause skin damage

15. Ensure that the patient is comfortable post the procedure

16. Dispose of all waste, including gloves and apron in the appropriate waste bags and clean any none disposable items according to correct procedures

17. Decontaminate hands according to correct hand hygiene techniques

18. Record the procedure in the patients records

74. Aseptic Technique: Wound Dressing Guidelines

Equipment

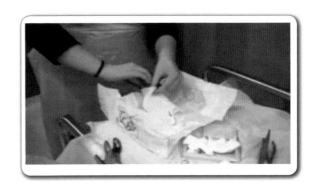

- Dressing Trolley

- Sterile dressing pack with contents

- Sterile 0.9% NACL for cleaning

- Hypoallergenic tape

- Appropriate dressings as required

- Alcohol hand-rub

- Any extra equipment e.g. sterile scissors

- Detergent wipe for cleaning trolley

Procedure

1. Check that all the equipment required for the procedure is available, and where applicable is sterile, dry and intact.

2. Explain and discuss the procedure with the patient and gain informed consent

3. Decontaminate hands using appropriate hand hygiene techniques. Alcohol hand-rub is the most appropriate method for hand hygiene during a procedure as long as hands are physically clean. Hands must be cleaned before and after every patient contact and before commencing the preparation for aseptic technique to prevent cross infection

4. Clean the trolley with detergent and water or disposable detergent wipes and dry with paper towel or use disposable wipes saturated with 70% isopropyl alcohol and leave to dry

5. Place the equipment on the bottom shelf of the clean dressing trolley

6. Position the patient comfortably on the couch/bed

7. Wearing gown and gloves loosen the adhesive on the old dressing

8. Clean hands with alcohol hand-rub

9. Open the outer cover of the sterile dressing pack and slide the contents without touching them onto the top shelf of the trolley

10. Open the sterile field using only the corners of the paper

11. Open any other packs, tipping their contents gently onto the centre of the sterile field

12. Where appropriate loosen the old dressing

13. Clean hands with alcohol hand-rub

14. Carefully lift the plastic disposable bag from the sterile field and using it as a sterile glove arrange the contents of the dressing pack and any other sterile items on the sterile field

15. With your hand enclosed within the sterile bag remove the old dressing from the wound. Invert the bag so that the dressing is contained within it and stick it to the trolley below the top shelf. This is the disposal bag for the remainder of the procedure for any waste other than sharps

16. Pour any solutions into gallipots or onto the intended plastic tray

17. Don the sterile gloves and carry out the dressing according to guidelines

18. Make sure the patient is comfortable post the procedure

19. Dispose of clinical waste and apron and gloves in the correct clinical waste bags

20. Clean the dressing trolley using correct technique

21. Clean hands with alcohol hand-rub or soap and water following correct hand hygiene techniques

22. Document the procedure clearly, including details of any dressings or devices used

Source: Dougherty, L. & Lister, S. (2015) The Royal Marsden Hospital Manual of Clinical Nursing Procedures. 9th Ed. Wiley Blackwell Pub: Chichester

75. Simple Wound Suturing Guidelines Interrupted Sutures

Equipment

- Dressing trolley
- Suture pack
- Sutures in varying gauges and materials
- 1% lidocaine hydrochloride
- 10 ml syringe (Sterile)
- Needles 21 and 25 G (Sterile)
- Sterile 0.9% NACL
- Dressings
- Plastic apron
- Sterile gloves
- Disposable razor
- Light source

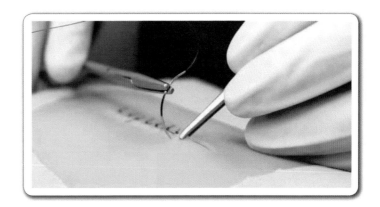

Procedure

1. Explain the procedure to the patient and gain informed consent
2. Ensure privacy, and that the patient is positioned comfortably on a trolley/ couch
3. Set up the dressing trolley with the equipment, and position close to the patient
4. To reduce the risk for contamination, follow the procedure for aseptic techniques (see separate guidelines for aseptic techniques)
5. Using a bright light, assess the wound, clean if necessary with sterile 0.9% NACL and decide the type of suture material and gauge of needle to use
6. The skin around the wound may require clipping to remove hair
7. Draw up the local anaesthetic and first administer an intra-cutaneous bleb using a fine needle. Wait for this to take effect, then inject the remainder through the anaesthetized area, infiltrating deeper using a longer, larger needle. Keep the point moving as injecting to ensure the needle is not in a blood vessel

8. Wait a minimum of 4-5 minutes and test the area for numbness with a needle tip prior to beginning. Do not begin the procedure until the anaesthetic has had time to act

9. Select appropriate tissue forceps, needle and needle holder

10. The needle should be grasped, in the needle holder on its flattened area about a third of the way along from the suture material

11. The needle holder should be held in the dominant hand and support the wound edge with the closed tips of tissue forceps

12. If a linear wound, suturing should begin at the centre

13. The needle should be inserted at a 90 degree angle to the skin and traverse the full thickness of the wound. The distance of the needle puncture from the edge of the wound should be equal to the depth of the layer of tissue being sutured. This does not apply to deep wounds where layered closure is required

14. Bring the needle up in between the wound edges

15. Pull the suture through the tissue until a short tail of approximately 2cm remains at the initial skin entry site

16. To bring the wound edges together, reinsert the needle at a 90 degree angle from the base of the wound on the other side and push the suture through the tissue, following the curve of the needle, so as to emerge perpendicular to the skin

17. To begin to create a knot hold the needle parallel to the skin, and grasping the needle end of the suture, make two clockwise loops around the needle holder to produce a surgeons knot

18. Grasp the tail of the suture with the needle holder. The wrapped suture will slide off the holder to encircle the tail

19. Pull the tail end of the suture towards you and the long suture strand away from you, making sure the suture lies flat

20. Follow this by a single anticlockwise loop around the needle holder and move the needle to the opposite side of the wound

21. Then create a third throw of one loop. Do not tie it too tightly, just enough to secure the knot

22. The suture can then be cut free from the knot, leaving tails of about 5mm

23. Insert each suture in the same way until the wound is entirely closed. The distance between adjacent sutures should be the same as the depth and width of each one

24. Once completed discard the needle in the sharps bin. Clean any blood from the surrounding area using aseptic technique and sterile 0.9% NACL

25. Apply a suitable dressing

26. Ensure the patient is comfortable post procedure and discuss care of the wound and follow up for suture removal

27. Dispose of all disposable sharps in the sharp bin and other waste including apron and gloves in the clinical waste bags. Clean the dressing trolley and other re-usable equipment according to correct techniques

28. Decontaminate hands according to correct hand hygiene techniques

29. Record the procedure in the patients notes, including date, time, name of practitioner, amount of local anaesthetic used, size and type of suture material and number of sutures

Source: Dougherty, L. & Lister, S. (2015) The Royal Marsden Hospital Manual of Clinical Nursing Procedures. 9th Ed. Wiley Blackwell Pub: Chichester

76. Suture Removal Guidelines

Equipment

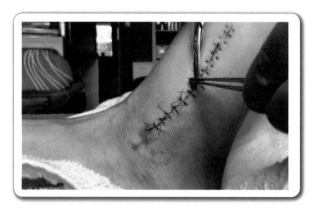

- Dressing trolley
- Sterile dressing pack
- Sterile stitch cutter or scissors
- Apron
- Gloves
- 0.9% NACL
- Metal forceps (sterile)
- Dressings (if required)
- Steristrips (if required)

Procedure

1. Explain the procedure to the patient and gain informed consent
2. Position patient comfortably in a chair or on the couch
3. Perform procedure using aseptic techniques
4. Decontaminate hands using correct hand hygiene procedure
5. Apply apron and gloves
6. Open the dressing pack and equipment onto a clean dressing trolley
7. To prevent infection clean the wound with 0.9% NACL
8. Using the forceps, lift the loose end of the suture, next to the knot
9. Metal forceps work better, as plastic forceps tend to slip against the nylon suture
10. Pull gently upwards and away from the skin

11. Insert the stitch cutter or scissors under one end of the suture and cut the stitch close to the skin

12. Gently pull the suture out

13. Continually assess the wound integrity throughout the procedure

14. For intermittent sutures alternate sutures should be removed first before remaining sutures are removed. Check that removed sutures are intact

15. Apply a suitable dressing or steri-strips to the wound (if required)

16. Dispose of disposable sharps in the sharps bin, and all clinical waste in appropriate waste/clinical waste bags.

17. Clean reusable equipment properly following manufacturers recommendations

18. Remove gloves and decontaminate hands adhering to correct hand hygiene techniques

19. Document the procedure in the patients notes and report any abnormal findings

Source: Dougherty, L. & Lister, S. (2015) The Royal Marsden Hospital Manual of Clinical Nursing Procedures. 9th Ed. Wiley Blackwell Pub: Chichester

77. Wound Clip/Staple Removal Guidelines

Equipment

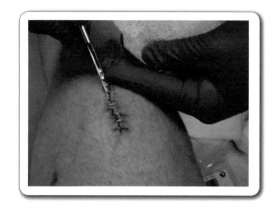

- Dressing trolley
- Sterile dressing pack
- Clip/ staple remover
- Apron
- Gloves
- 0.9% NACL
- Dressings (if required)
- Steristrips (if required)

Procedure

1. Explain the procedure to the patient and gain informed consent

2. Position patient comfortably in a chair or on the couch

3. Perform procedure using aseptic techniques

4. Decontaminate hands using correct hand hygiene procedure

5. Apply apron and gloves

6. Remove dressing and inspect the wound. After assessing the wound, determine if the wound is sufficiently healed to have the staples/clips removed

7. Open the dressing pack and equipment onto a clean dressing trolley

8. Prepare the sterile field and add necessary supplies (clip/ staple remover)

9. To prevent infection clean the wound with 0.9% NACL. This reduces the risk of infection from microorganisms on the wound site or surrounding skin. Cleaning also loosens and removes any dried blood or crusted exudate from the staples/ clips and wound bed

10. Continually assess the wound integrity throughout the procedure

11. Place lower tip of clip/ staple remover beneath the staple. Do not pull up while depressing handle on staple remover or change the angle of your wrist or hand. Close the handle, then gently move the staple side to side to remove

12. When both ends of the clip/staple are visible, move the staple remover away from the skin and place the clip/staple on a sterile piece of gauze by releasing the handles on the staple remover

13. Continue to remove every second staple to the end of the incision line. Alternating removal of staples provides strength to incision line while removing staples and prevents accidental separation of incision line

14. Apply a suitable dressing and or steri-strips to the wound (if required)

15. Place steri-strips on location of every removed staple along incision line if required

16. Apply a sterile dressing on the incision site or leave exposed to air if the wound is not irritated

17. Dispose of all disposable sharps in the sharps bin, and all clinical waste in appropriate waste/ clinical waste bags

18. Clean the dressing trolley and any reusable equipment properly following manufacturers guidelines

19. Remove gloves and decontaminate hands adhering to correct hand hygiene techniques

20. Document the procedure in the patients notes and report any problems with the wound or abnormal findings

Source: Dougherty, L. & Lister, S. (2015) The Royal Marsden Hospital Manual of Clinical Nursing Procedures. 9th Ed. Wiley Blackwell Pub: Chichester.

78. Tissue Adhesive (Glue) for Minor Laceration Guidelines

Indications for use

Tissue adhesive/ glue is an acceptable alternative to standard wound closure for repairing simple traumatic lacerations, specifically:

- Closure of minor skin wounds (usually less than 3 cm in length)
- Low-tension wounds on the scalp, face, trunk and limbs
- Clean wounds with easily-aligned edges

Equipment

- Sterile dressing pack

- Sterile gauze

- Sterile 0.9% sodium chloride for wound cleansing

- Gloves

- Tissue adhesive (Glue)

- Steri-strips

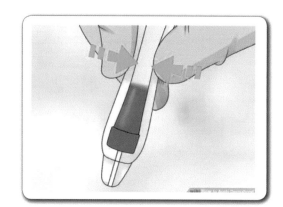

Procedure

1. Explain the procedure to the patient and gain informed consent

2. Position the patient comfortably on the bed/couch

3. Decontaminate hands according to correct hand hygiene techniques

4. Open the dressing pack and prepare all equipment for the procedure using an aseptic non-touch technique

5. Holding the container with the nozzle uppermost, flick the tip of the tissue adhesive ampoule

6. Twist and remove the cap to open the vial (retain the cap until procedure is completed)

7. Attach the fine tip precision cannula (applicator) to the ampoule with a twisting motion

8. Conduct the procedure using an aseptic non-touch technique

9. Check the wound for foreign bodies and remove any if present

10. Clean and dry the wound thoroughly and ensure the area is free from excessive blood

11. Ensure that wound edges appose readily

12. Hold the wound edges together with fingers, forceps or other appropriate method and apply adhesive sparingly, as a very thin film along the length of the wound, either intermittently or in a continuous line. Light pressure is sufficient to express the tissue adhesive. Avoid adhesive entering the wound

13. Continue to hold the wound edges together with light pressure for 30 seconds or until the adhesive is dry

14. Steri-strips may also be applied to the wound (no secondary dressing is necessary)

15. Remove the fine tip precision cannula (applicator) with a twisting motion and re-fit the reversed winged cap to the ampoule. Dispose of the applicator and ampoule to the sharps bin or clinical waste

16. Dispose of all waste appropriately in correct waste and clinical waste bins

17. Decontaminate hands according to correct hand hygiene techniques

18. Ensure patient is comfortable post procedure and that aftercare advice is given

19. Record the procedure in the patients notes, detailing the procedure and the condition of the wound

Source: : Our Lady's Hospital, Crumlin (2012). Nursing Practice Committee Guidelines on the Use of Tissue Adhesive for Minor Laceration Repair. OLCHC: Dublin.

79. Wound Swab Sampling Guidelines

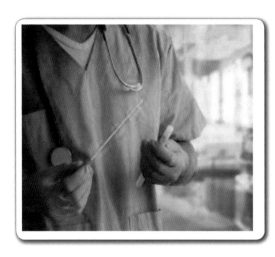

Equipment

- Non sterile gloves
- Apron
- Sterile swabs (bacterial or viral) with transport medium
- Microbiology request forms
- 0.9% NACL
- Dressing pack containing sterile gloves and dressings

Procedure

1. Explain the procedure to the patient and gain informed consent
2. Set up the equipment
3. Decontaminate hands using correct hand hygiene procedure
4. Position patient comfortably
5. Apply apron and gloves
6. Remove current dressing if applicable and dispose in clinical waste
7. Remove gloves and decontaminate hands. Open sterile dressing pack, decant sterile swab and don sterile gloves
8. Remove swab from outer packaging
9. Rotate the swab tip over a 1cm area of viable tissue, or at the near centre of the wound for 5 seconds, applying enough pressure to express tissue fluid from the wound bed

10. If the wound is dry, the tip of the swab should be moistened with 0.9% sodium chloride

11. If pus is present, it should be aspirated using a sterile syringe and decanted into a sterile specimen pot

12. Remove cap from the transport tube. Carefully place swab in the transport tube, ensuring it is fully immersed in the transport medium. Ensure cap is firmly secured

13. Redress the wound (if applicable) as per care plan

14. Discard waste in appropriate waste containers, remove gloves and apron and decontaminate hands according to correct hand hygiene techniques

15. Complete the microbiology request form with patient details, including relevant information such as exact site, nature of specimen and investigation required. Arrange delivery to Lab (Keep at room temperature)

16. Document the procedure in the patients notes

80. Wound Drain Removal Guidelines

Equipment

- Dressing trolley
- Dressing pack
- 0.9% NACL
- Sterile stitch cutter
- Protective apron
- Sterile swabs
- Non-sterile gloves
- Sterile gloves
- Adhesive/ hypoallergenic tape
- Sterile disposable forceps X 2

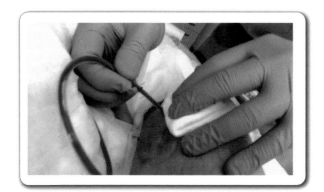

Procedure

1. Explain and discuss the procedure with the patient and gain informed consent
2. Decontaminate hands adhering to correct hand hygiene techniques
3. Wear a protective apron and disposable gloves
4. Set up the trolley and prepare equipment ready for use
5. Ensure privacy and that the patient is in a comfortable position, which allows access to the suture(s) securing the drain
6. Loosen dressing around drain
7. If vacuum drain in situ, loosen connection at drain bottle to break vacuum
8. Clamp drain tube with plastic clamp (attached to tubing)
9. Decontaminate hands adhering to correct hand hygiene techniques and put on sterile gloves
10. With one set of forceps, the loose dressing should be removed, and dressing and forceps disposed
11. Observe skin surrounding the drain site for signs of excoriation, oedema, infection or purulent exudate

12. If drain site appears inflamed or purulent a swab should be taken and sent for microbiology and sensitivity

13. The skin surrounding the drain site should only be cleaned with NACL 0.9% if necessary, i.e. the drain site is purulent or to ensure the suture is visible and accessible

14. Using a non-touch technique place a sterile field/sheet under drain

15. Using remaining forceps, lift the loose end of the suture, next to the knot and pull gently

16. Insert the stitch cutter under one end of the suture and cut

17. Gently pull the suture out, ensuring external suture material is not pulled through the wound

18. Using sterile swabs grip the wound drain in one hand and place sterile swabs over the drain entry site

19. Gently pull the wound drain and apply gentle support at the entry site

20. Continue pulling the drain until removed

21. Document amount and nature of drainage and dispose as clinical waste

22. Reassure the patient and inform of procedure at each stage

23. Inspect drain site and remove any exudate with a dry sterile swab

24. Cover with a sterile dressing and secure with tape

25. Dispose of sharps in the sharps bin and all clinical waste in clinical waste bins. Clean all reusable equipment properly following manufacturers recommendations

26. Decontaminate hands adhering to correct hand hygiene techniques

27. Document procedure and report any abnormal findings

Source: Dougherty, L. & Lister, S. (2015) The Royal Marsden Hospital Manual of Clinical Nursing Procedures. 9th Ed. Wiley Blackwell Pub: Chichester.

81. Motivating Behavioural Change in Clients

The Transtheoretical Model

The Transtheoretical Model or Wheel of Change, proposed by the Psychologists James Prochaska and Carlo Di-Clemente helps people make behavioural changes and can be used for structured motivational therapy interventions in practice. The model is particularly helpful in situations where a client is trying to break an addictive behaviour. It can be applied to a range of habitual problems, including:

- Smoking
- Misuse of alcohol/ drugs
- Eating problems
- Other addictive behaviours

The Transtheoretical Model /Wheel of Change

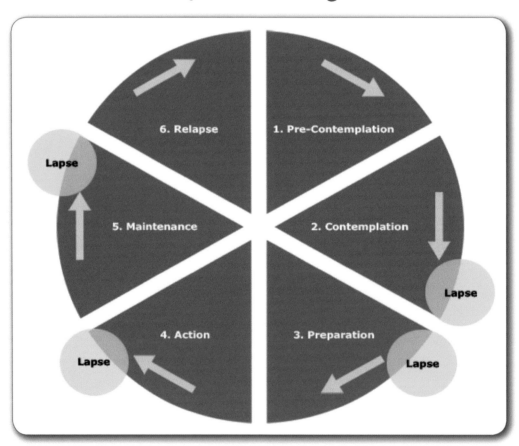

82. Motivating Behavioural Change in Clients

Stages of Change

Pre-contemplation Stage

- No interest in changing the behaviour

- Personal advantages

- Has mostly positive thoughts about the behaviour

Contemplation Stage

- Aware of some personal disadvantages

- Thinking about changing some aspects of the behaviour

- Still has some reasons for continuing the behaviour

Preparation Stage

- Intending to make a change

- Knows why they want to change

- Planning when and how to do it

Action

- Believing that change is possible

- Making an attempt to change

Maintenance

- Behaviour change is ongoing

- Able to cope without relapsing

- Support and encouragement

Relapse

This attempt is unsuccessful Returns to one of the above stages

It is common to go through various stages 3-4 times before reaching the maintenance stage, hence its name –the cycle of change or wheel of change. Passing through this cycle will take time, which can be months or years depending on individual circumstances.

Stage	Possible Strategies
Pre-Contemplation	
Client not considering change and may be presenting with challenging behaviours.	Non-judgemental, provide information in a non-authoritarian way, use of unconditional positive regard, reinforce the client's potential to change.
Stage 1- Contemplation	
Client has begun to see some benefits in changing but has not yet resolved to change	1. Support client to evaluate the pros and cons of making change. 2. Help the client to look at the various options available to them and the possible effects e.g. stopping altogether / cutting down / joining a support group. 3. Are they small ways the client can begin to step towards change?
Stage 2 - Action	
Client has resolved to make changes but may be unsure how to proceed and may be fearful / nervous.	1. At this point, introduce the model to the client as a visual aid. 2. Support the client to plan change rather than rushing into it. 3. Support the client in goal-setting (SMART). 4. Support the client in drawing up a commitment to change. 5. Reinforce the benefits of changing. 6. Explore other support options for the client e.g. a local support group / leisure activities / new hobby.
Stage 3 - Action	
Client has committed to change and works to try and achieve it.	1. Support the client in following their plan and monitoring and reviewing the progress. 2. Acknowledge successes (even small ones) and encourage the client to reward themselves. 3. Reinforce the benefits of change and help the client to identify these benefits as they occur. 4. Acknowledge the client in a holistic way i.e. their life outside their plan for change, help them to factor in time to unwind without focusing on their plan. 5. Help the client to recognize and learn from strategies that aren't working and identify alternatives. 6. If a lapse occurs, use the model to show how much progress they have made and emphasise that they are not going back to square one.
Stage 4 - Maintenance	
Client moves into maintaining the change that they have made successfully	1. At this stage, recognizing that change is an ongoing process is important –the client's problem may never fully go away, but they are better able to manage and control it. 2. Monitoring and reviewing progress may still be helpful at this stage, use the model and plans until the client is ready to manage without them. 3. If a lapse occurs at this stage, again use the model to reinforce the progress already made. Support the client in considering why the lapse occurred so that they can learn from it. 4. Explore ways in which the client could help those in a similar situation; using their experience to

Stage	Possible Strategies
Lapse	
The client slips back to the problem behavior on one occasion, but is able to return to the plan without much difficulty.	1. Acknowledge that lapse is part of success and support the client in understanding the reasons for the lapse. 2. Help the client to plan alternative ways of managing in similar situations in the future. 3. Reinforce and build on the progress already made.
Relapse	
The client slips back to the problem behavior for a prolonged period, and finds it very difficult to get back on track.	1. Again, acknowledge that relapse is part of success and can be a learning opportunity. 2. The client may need to return to the "Decision" or even "Contemplation" stage of the model, however it is still important to recognize the progress made up to the point of relapse. 3. Support the client in re-working their plan of action and learning from their relapse.

References

Prochaska, J.O. & DiClemente, C.C (1982). 'Trans-theoretical Therapy: Towards a More Integrative Model of Change' *Psychotherapy: Research, Theory & Practice* 19(3) pp.276-288.

Prochaska, J.O., DiClemente, C.C & Norcross, J.C. (1992). 'In Search of How People Change: Applications to Addictive Behaviours' *American Psychologist* 47 (9) pp.1102-1114.

83. Brief Interventions for Smoking Cessation

Brief interventions are a range of effective behaviour change interventions that are client centred, short in duration and used in a variety of settings by health and other professionals. They use an empathic approach, emphasising self-efficacy and personal responsibility for change, information giving and details of resources available to support change.

For smoking cessation, brief interventions involve opportunistic advice, discussion, negotiation and encouragement that typically take between 5 and 10 minutes. The intervention may involve referral to a more intensive treatment if appropriate. Interventions should be recorded and followed up as appropriate.

Brief Intervention for Smoking Cessation

The 5 A's
The five components of the Framework are:

1. **Ask**
   Systematically identify all smokers at every visit. Record smoking status, no. of cigarettes smoked per day/week and year started smoking.

2. **Advise**
   Urge all smokers to quit. Advice should be clear and personalised.

3. **Assess**
   Determine willingness and confidence to make a quit attempt; note the stage of change.

4. **Assist**
   Aid the smoker in quitting. Provide behavioural support. Recommend/prescribe pharmacological aids. If not ready to quit promote motivation for future attempt.

5. **Arrange**
   Follow-up appointment within 1 week or if appropriate refer to specialist cessation service for intensive support. Document the intervention.

References
Health Service Executive (2012). Brief Intervention for Smoking Cessation National Training Programme. Participant Resource. HSE: Dublin

Weight Management Treatment Algorithm

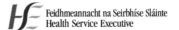 Feidhmeannacht na Seirbhíse Sláinte Health Service Executive

A Quick Reference Guide For Primary Care Staff

(See www.icgp.ie/weightmanagement or www.hse.ie for additional online resources)

Raising the issue

> "I haven't checked your weight & height in a while. I can check it today as part of your check up? "

> "Do you think your weight (or general lifestyle) may be contributing to your back pain/fertility problem/ arthritis/reflux/diabetes/BP?"

If patient agrees to engage proceed to assessment or arrange next appointment. The exercise & food diary could be given at this stage.

(www.icgp.ie/ weightmanagement)

If patient is not keen to engage do not push the issue but offer to revisit it at a later date.

Initial assessment

> BMI 18.5 – 25.0 reassure and advise re ongoing self-monitoring. (If BMI < 18.5 consider appropriate referral)

> BMI 25.0 – 40.0

- Assess readiness to change

- Assess patient's expectation & agree realistic target weight loss of 5 – 10% over 6 months.

> Show patient the category they are in on BMI chart (www.icgp.ie/weightmanagement).

> Advise of benefits of 10% weight loss

> Advise patient to keep a food & exercise diary for 4 days (www.icgp.ie/weightmanagement)

> BMI > 40 proceed with above and arrange referral to hospital based weight management service. (www.icgp.ie/weightmanagement)

Benefits of a 10% loss in presenting body weight

> 37% reduction in cancer deaths

> 20% reduction in all cause mortality,

> 40% reduction in diabetes related mortality

> 10mmHg reduction in systolic BP

> Improved lipid profile

> Improved fertility

> Improved mood & self-confidence

 Stress that "obesity" is a clinical term with health implications, rather than a question of how one looks.

Relevant History

> Medical history – relevant co-morbidities: diabetes, cardiovascular disease, cancer, operative history, PCOS, GORD, sleep apnoea, sub fertility, back pain, osteoarthritis, depression, medications & family history.

> Weight history (onset & progression of weight gain, peak weight)

> Dieting history (previous attempts, what diets, what worked, lowest weight achieved, reason for regaining weight)

> Physical activity history: objectify time spent (minutes per week); walk/cycle including transport to work (walk, cycle Vs car), leisure exercise (swim, golf, walk dog, etc.)

> Physical inactivity history: objectify time spent (minutes per week); watching TV & computer, in car, prolonged sedentary periods.

> Food intake i.e. home cooked/processed/take away, high carbohydrates/fats/sugar/salt, portion sizes, snacks, alcohol, supermarket habits – multipacks of bars/crisps etc.

> Psychological history – history of depression, anxiety or eating disorders. (See www.icgp.ie/weightmanagement for screening tools)

Source: Irish College of General Practitioners (2017). HSE/ICGP Weight Management Treatment Algorithm for Adults. ICGP: Dublin

Physical Activity (P.A.) Guidelines
www.getirelandactive.ie

Suggest starting with <u>small, regular, planned</u> bouts of P.A. (10 minutes or less). Build to target time over months.

Weight maintenance

> Suggest 30 – 60 minutes moderate intensity P.A. between 5 to 7 days a week (> 150 mins per week)

> 60 minutes of moderate or 30 minutes of vigorous activity per day

> This can be broken up into smaller cumulative blocks (e.g. 15 mins x 5, 25 mins x 3, 35 mins x 2)

To lose weight

> Suggest 60 – 75 minutes of moderate intensity P.A. per day between 5 to 7 days a week (> 250 mins per week)

BMI > 40 Grade III
- Severe Obesity
- High Risk
- Specialist Referral indicated

BMI > 30 Obese or Very Obese
- Combination of Diet, physical activity, psychology + or - pharmacotherapy

BMI > 25-30 with co-morbidities
- Advise patient re health risks
- Highlight need for lifestyle change to revert to a healthy weight

BMI > 25 patient overweight or obese
- Assess readiness to change and proceed

Calculate BMI regularly and advise patient accordingly

BMI < 18.5 Refer if appropriate	BMI 18.5 – 25 **Healthy Weight**	BMI 25 – 30 **Overweight**	BMI 25 – 30 + Co-morbidities **Overweight**	BMI 30 – 35 **Grade I Obesity**	BMI 35 – 40 **Grade II Very Obese**	BMI > 40 **Grade III Severe Obesity**

> *Stress that consistent weight loss of 0.5 -1kg (1-2lbs) per week will result in reaching the target weight of 10% weight loss.*

Subsequent visits / referral options

> Recheck BMI and assess trend

> Assess the food & exercise diary - identify & agree areas for improvement (www.icgp.ie/weightmanagement). Reset target.

> Explore any contributing factors i.e. medical & social, family & environmental factors.

> Consider referral to a Dietitian, Physiotherapist/Physical Activity Specialist or Psychologist. Referrals where possible should be within the Primary Care Team/Network to maximize multidisciplinary management.

> Refer to the GP Exercise Referral Programme/Green Prescription, if available in your area, or advise re regular, planned exercise. Emphasise self-monitoring of time involved (minutes per week). Use Physical Activity Diary. (www.icgp.ie/weightmanagement)

> Reweigh & explain that weight loss may be slow (or absent) in initial weeks but persistence will achieve results. Explore reasons for lack of weight loss.

> Consider referral to commercial, self-help & community organisations e.g. Weight Watchers & Unislim, as well as the online resource www.safefood.eu/weigh2live all of which are evidence based.

> Agree regular follow up – ideally every 4 weeks.

> Once 10% weight loss is achieved encourage weight maintenance for 6 months

> Consider other options e.g. pharmacotherapy (see box), bariatric surgery (hospital referral for BMI >40) (www.icgp.ie/weightmanagement)

Pharmacotherapy

Only one agent is currently licensed for the treatment of obesity – Orlistat. It is hoped that other agents will become available soon.

Orlistat

> Prescribe only as part of an overall plan for managing obesity in adults who have:
- BMI of 28.0 kg/m2 or more with associated risk factors,
  Or
- BMI of 30.0 kg/m2 or more.

> Continue treatment for longer than 3 months only if the person has lost at least 5% of their initial body weight since starting drug treatment (less strict with type 2 diabetics).

> Continue for longer than 12 months (usually for weight maintenance) only after discussing potential benefits and limitations with the patient.

Contraceptive renewal

> Advise patient that oestrogen containing contraceptives are not advised with BMI > 39 due to increased CV & thromboembolic risk.

> For BMI 30 – 39 advise patient of importance of weight loss, both for reduced cardiovascular risk and improved fertility.

> Consider alternatives & record.

Source: Irish College of General Practitioners (2017). BMI Chart for use with the Weight Management Treatment Algorithm for Adults. ICGP: Dublin

BMI Chart (Kgs/m²) for use with the Weight Management Treatment Algorithm

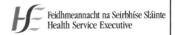

A Quick Reference Guide For Primary Care Staff
(See www.icgp.ie/weightmanagement or www.hse.ie for additional online resources)

Underweight (<18.5 kgs/m²)		Healthy weight (18.5 -24.9 kgs/m²)			Overweight (25 - 29.9 kgs/m²)			Obese Class I (30 - 34.9 kgs/m²)			Obese Class II (35 - 39.9 kgs/m²)			Obese Class III (> 40 kgs/m²)		

Stone	lbs	4'10"	4'11"	5'0"	5'1"	5'2"	5'3"	5'4"	5'5"	5'6"	5'7"	5'8"	5'9"	5'10"	5'11"	6'0"	6'1"	6'2"	6'3"	kgs
7st 2lbs	100	20.9	20.2	19.6	18.9	18.3	17.8	17.2	16.7	16.2	15.7	15.2	14.8	14.4	14.0	13.6	13.2	12.9	12.5	45.5 kgs
7st 7lbs	105	22.0	21.3	20.5	19.9	19.2	18.6	18.1	17.5	17.0	16.5	16.0	15.5	15.1	14.7	14.3	13.9	13.5	13.2	47.7 kgs
7st 12lbs	110	23.0	22.3	21.5	20.8	20.2	19.5	18.9	18.3	17.8	17.3	16.8	16.3	15.8	15.4	14.9	14.5	14.2	13.8	50 kgs
8st 3lbs	115	24.1	23.3	22.5	21.8	21.1	20.4	19.8	19.2	18.6	18.0	17.5	17.0	16.5	16.1	15.6	15.2	14.8	14.4	52.3 kgs
8st 8lbs	120	25.1	24.3	23.5	22.7	22.0	21.3	20.6	20.0	19.4	18.8	18.3	17.8	17.3	16.8	16.3	15.9	15.4	15.0	54.5 kgs
8st 13lbs	125	26.2	25.3	24.5	23.7	22.9	22.2	21.5	20.8	20.2	19.6	19.0	18.4	18.0	17.5	17.0	16.5	16.1	15.7	56.8 kgs
9st 4lbs	130	27.2	26.3	25.4	24.6	23.8	23.1	22.4	21.7	21.0	20.4	19.8	19.2	18.7	18.2	17.7	17.2	16.7	16.3	59.1 kgs
9st 9lbs	135	28.3	27.3	26.4	25.6	24.7	24.0	23.2	22.5	21.8	21.2	20.6	20.0	19.4	18.9	18.3	17.8	17.4	16.9	61.4 kgs
10st 0lbs	140	29.3	28.3	27.4	26.5	25.7	24.9	24.1	23.3	22.6	22.0	21.3	20.7	20.1	19.6	19.0	18.5	18.0	17.5	63.6 kgs
10st 5lbs	145	30.4	29.3	28.4	27.5	26.6	25.7	24.9	24.2	23.5	22.8	22.1	21.5	20.8	20.3	19.7	19.2	18.7	18.2	65.9 kgs
10st 10lbs	150	31.4	30.4	29.4	28.4	27.5	26.6	25.8	25.0	24.3	23.5	22.9	22.2	21.6	21.0	20.4	19.8	19.3	18.8	68.2 kgs
11st 1lbs	155	32.5	31.4	30.3	29.3	28.4	27.5	26.7	25.8	25.1	24.3	23.6	22.9	22.3	21.7	21.1	20.5	19.9	19.4	70.5 kgs
11st 6lbs	160	33.5	32.4	31.3	30.3	29.3	28.4	27.5	26.7	25.9	25.1	24.4	23.7	23.0	22.4	21.7	21.2	20.6	20.0	72.7 kgs
11st 11lbs	165	34.6	33.4	32.3	31.2	30.2	29.3	28.4	27.5	26.7	25.9	25.1	24.4	23.7	23.1	22.4	21.8	21.2	20.7	75 kgs
12st 2lbs	170	35.6	34.4	33.3	32.2	31.2	30.2	29.2	28.3	27.5	26.7	25.9	25.2	24.4	23.8	23.1	22.5	21.9	21.3	77.3 kgs
12st 7lbs	175	36.7	35.4	34.2	33.1	32.1	31.1	30.1	29.2	28.3	27.5	26.7	25.9	25.2	24.5	23.8	23.1	22.5	21.9	79.5 kgs
12st 12lbs	180	37.7	36.4	35.2	34.1	33.0	32.0	31.0	30.0	29.1	28.3	27.4	26.6	25.9	25.2	24.5	23.8	23.2	22.5	81.8 kgs
13st 3lbs	185	38.7	37.4	36.2	35.0	33.9	32.8	31.8	30.8	29.9	29.0	28.2	27.4	26.6	25.9	25.1	24.5	23.8	23.2	84.1 kgs
13st 8lbs	190	39.8	38.5	37.2	36.0	34.8	33.7	32.7	31.7	30.7	29.8	28.9	28.1	27.3	26.6	25.8	25.1	24.4	23.8	86.4 kgs
13st 13lbs	195	40.8	39.5	38.2	36.9	35.7	34.6	33.5	32.5	31.5	30.6	29.7	28.9	28.0	27.3	26.5	25.8	25.1	24.4	88.6 kgs
14st 4lbs	200	41.9	40.5	39.1	37.9	36.7	35.5	34.4	33.4	32.3	31.4	30.5	29.6	28.8	28.0	27.2	26.4	25.7	25.1	90.9 kgs
14st 9lbs	205	42.9	41.5	40.1	38.8	37.6	36.4	35.3	34.2	33.2	32.2	31.2	30.3	29.5	28.7	27.9	27.1	26.4	25.7	93.2 kgs
15st 0lbs	210	44.0	42.5	41.1	39.8	38.5	37.3	36.1	35.0	34.0	33.0	32.0	31.1	30.2	29.4	28.5	27.8	27.0	26.3	95.5 kgs
15st 5lbs	215	45.0	43.5	42.1	40.7	39.4	38.2	37.0	35.9	34.8	33.7	32.8	31.8	30.9	30.0	29.2	28.4	27.7	26.9	97.7 kgs
15st 10lbs	220	46.1	44.5	43.1	41.7	40.3	39.1	37.8	36.7	35.6	34.5	33.5	32.6	31.6	30.7	29.9	29.1	28.3	27.6	100 kgs
16st 1lbs	225	47.1	45.5	44.0	42.6	41.2	39.9	38.7	37.5	36.4	35.3	34.3	33.3	32.4	31.4	30.6	29.7	28.9	28.2	102.3 kgs
16st 6lbs	230	48.2	46.6	45.0	43.5	42.2	40.8	39.6	38.4	37.2	36.1	35.0	34.0	33.1	32.1	31.3	30.4	29.6	28.8	104.5 kgs
16st 11lbs	235	49.2	47.6	46.0	44.5	43.1	41.7	40.4	39.2	38.0	36.9	35.8	34.8	33.8	32.8	31.9	31.1	30.2	29.4	106.8 kgs
17st 2lbs	240	50.3	48.6	47.0	45.4	44.0	42.6	41.3	40.0	38.8	37.7	36.6	35.5	34.5	33.5	32.6	31.7	30.9	30.1	109.1 kgs
17st 7lbs	245	51.3	49.6	47.9	46.4	44.9	43.5	42.1	40.9	39.6	38.5	37.3	36.3	35.2	34.2	33.3	32.4	31.5	30.7	111.4 kgs
17st 12lbs	250	52.4	50.6	48.9	47.3	45.8	44.4	43.0	41.7	40.4	39.2	38.1	37.0	35.9	34.9	34.0	33.1	32.2	31.3	113.6 kgs
18st 3lbs	255	53.4	51.6	49.9	48.3	46.7	45.3	43.9	42.5	41.2	40.0	38.9	37.7	36.7	35.6	34.7	33.7	32.8	31.9	115.9 kgs
18st 8lbs	260	54.5	52.6	50.9	49.2	47.7	46.2	44.7	43.4	42.1	40.8	39.6	38.5	37.4	36.3	35.3	34.4	33.5	32.6	118.2 kgs
18st 13lbs	265	55.5	53.6	51.9	50.2	48.6	47.0	45.6	44.2	42.9	41.6	40.4	39.2	38.1	37.0	36.0	35.0	34.1	33.2	120.5 kgs
19st 4lbs	270	56.5	54.6	52.8	51.1	49.5	47.9	46.4	45.0	43.7	42.4	41.1	40.0	38.8	37.7	36.7	35.7	34.7	33.8	122.7 kgs
19st 9lbs	275	57.6	55.7	53.8	52.1	50.4	48.8	47.3	45.9	44.5	43.2	41.9	40.7	39.5	38.4	37.4	36.4	35.4	34.4	125 kgs
20st 0lbs	280	58.6	56.7	54.8	53.0	51.3	49.7	48.2	46.7	45.3	43.9	42.7	41.4	40.3	39.1	38.1	37.0	36.0	35.1	127.3 kgs
20st 5lbs	285	59.7	57.7	55.8	54.0	52.2	50.6	49.0	47.5	46.1	44.7	43.4	42.2	41.0	39.8	38.7	37.7	36.7	35.7	129.5 kgs
20st 10lbs	290	60.7	58.7	56.8	54.9	53.2	51.5	49.9	48.4	46.9	45.5	44.2	42.9	41.7	40.5	39.4	38.3	37.3	36.3	131.8 kgs
21st 1lbs	295	61.8	59.7	57.7	55.9	54.1	52.4	50.7	49.2	47.7	46.3	44.9	43.7	42.4	41.2	40.1	39.0	38.0	36.9	134.1 kgs
21st 6lbs	300	62.8	60.7	58.7	56.8	55.0	53.3	51.6	50.0	48.5	47.1	45.7	44.4	43.1	41.9	40.8	39.7	38.6	37.6	136.4 kgs
21st 11lbs	305	63.9	61.7	59.7	57.7	55.9	54.1	52.5	50.9	49.3	47.9	46.5	45.1	43.9	42.6	41.5	40.3	39.2	38.2	138.6 kgs
22st 2lbs	310	64.9	62.7	60.7	58.7	56.8	55.0	53.3	51.7	50.1	48.7	47.2	45.9	44.6	43.3	42.1	41.0	39.9	38.8	140.9 kgs
22st 7lbs	315	66.0	63.8	61.6	59.6	57.7	55.9	54.2	52.5	50.9	49.4	48.0	46.6	45.3	44.0	42.8	41.6	40.5	39.5	143.2 kgs
22st 12lbs	320	67.0	64.8	62.6	60.6	58.7	56.8	55.0	53.4	51.8	50.2	48.8	47.4	46.0	44.7	43.5	42.3	41.2	40.1	145.5 kgs
23st 3lbs	325	68.1	65.8	63.6	61.5	59.6	57.7	55.9	54.2	52.6	51.0	49.5	48.1	46.7	45.4	44.2	43.0	41.8	40.7	147.7 kgs
23st 8lbs	330	69.1	66.8	64.6	62.5	60.5	58.6	56.8	55.0	53.4	51.8	50.3	48.8	47.4	46.1	44.8	43.6	42.5	41.3	150 kgs
23st 13lbs	335	70.2	67.8	65.6	63.4	61.4	59.5	57.6	55.9	54.2	52.6	51.0	49.6	48.2	46.8	45.5	44.3	43.1	42.0	152.3 kgs
24st 4lbs	340	71.2	68.8	66.5	64.4	62.3	60.4	58.5	56.7	55.0	53.4	51.8	50.3	48.9	47.5	46.2	45.0	43.7	42.6	154.5 kgs
24st 9lbs	345	72.3	69.8	67.5	65.3	63.2	61.2	59.3	57.5	55.8	54.1	52.6	51.1	49.6	48.2	46.9	45.6	44.4	43.2	156.8 kgs
25st 0lbs	350	73.3	70.8	68.5	66.3	64.1	62.1	60.2	58.4	56.6	54.9	53.3	51.8	50.3	48.9	47.6	46.3	45.0	43.8	159.1 kgs
25st 5lbs	355	74.4	71.9	69.5	67.2	65.1	63.0	61.1	59.2	57.4	55.7	54.1	52.5	51.0	49.6	48.2	46.9	45.7	44.5	161.4 kgs
		147.3 cms	149.9 cms	152.4 cms	154.9 cms	157.5 cms	160 cms	162.6 cms	165.1 cms	167.6 cms	170.2 cms	172.7 cms	175.3 cms	177.8 cms	180.3 cms	182.9 cms	185.4 cms	188 cms	190.5 cms	

Source: Irish College of General Practitioners (2017). HSE/ICGP Weight Management Treatment Algorithm for Adults. ICGP: Dublin

85. Childhood Immunisation Schedule Ireland

Birth - 13 months

Anaphylaxis pack

Epinephrine must be available when giving vaccines. See Anaphylaxis Guidelines

Age Months	Vaccinate	Type of Vaccination
At Birth		- BCG/Tuberculosis Vaccine (given in maternity hospitals or HSE clinic)
2	GP Surgery	- 6 in 1 Vaccine (Diphtheria Tetanus Whooping Cough (Pertussis) Hib (Haemophilus influenzae b) Polio (Inactivated poliomyelitis) Hepatitis B) - PCV (Pneumococcal Conjugate Vaccine) - MenB Vaccine (Meningococcal B Vaccine) - Rotavirus oral vaccine
4	GP Surgery	- 6 in 1 Vaccine (Diphtheria Tetanus Whooping Cough (Pertussis) Hib (Haemophilus influenzae typeb) Polio (Inactivated poliomyelitis) Hepatitis B) - MenB Vaccine (Meningococcal B Vaccine) - Rotavirus oral vaccine
6	GP Surgery	- 6 in 1 Vaccine (Diphtheria Tetanus Whooping Cough (Pertussis) Hib (Haemophilus influenzae b) Polio (Inactivated poliomyelitis) Hepatitis B) - PCV (Pneumococcal Conjugate Vaccine) - MenC Vaccine (Meningococcal C Vaccine)
12	GP Surgery	- MMR (Measles Mumps Rubella) - MenB Vaccine (Meningococcal B Vaccine)
13	GP Surgery	- Hib/MenC (Haemophilus influenzae b and Meningococcal C combined vaccine) - PCV (Pneumococcal Conjugate Vaccine)

Source: Refer to main HSE Immunisation Guidelines and HSE (2018). Guidelines for vaccination in General Practice. HSE National Immunisation Office: Dublin.

Recommended Childhood Immunisation schedule 2016

Age Months		Immunisations	Type of Comment
Birth		BCG*	1 injection
2 months		DTaP/Hib/IPV/Hep B + MenB +PCV + Rotavirus	3 injections+ oral vaccine
4 months		DTaP/Hib/IPV/Hep B+ MenB + Rotavirus	2 injections+ oral vaccine
6 months		DTaP/Hib/IPV/Hep B + PCV + MenC + Rotavirus	3 injections(+ oral vaccine)
12 months		MMR + MenB	2 injections
13 months		Hib / MenC/ + PCV	2 injections
4 - 5 years		DTaP/IPV** +MMR	2 injections
12-13 years	Girls	HPV (2 doses 6 months apart) Tdap, MenC	4 injections
	Boys	Tdap, MenC	2 injections

86. School Programme Immunisations Ireland

Protects against the following diseases with the named vaccines:

- Measles, mumps, rubella with MMR vaccine

- Tetanus, diphtheria, polio, pertussis with Tdap/IPV vaccine

- Low dose tetanus, diphtheria, low dose pertussis with Tdap vaccine

- Meningococcal C infection with MenC vaccine

- Human papillomavirus (HPV) with HPV vaccine

Recommended childhood vaccines given in schools immunisation programme are free

- 4 in 1 and MMR (Age 4-5)

- Tdap Programme (Age 12-13)

- MenC Programme (Age 12-13)

- HPV Programme (Age 12-13)

References
Health Service Executive (2018). School Programme Immunisations Schedule. HSE: Dublin

87. Guidelines Prior to Vaccination

1. Ensure that a GP is present in the building while vaccinations are being given and for 15 minutes after the last vaccine is administered to deal with anaphylaxis or any other adverse events that might occur, including syncope. Anaphylaxis Pack must be available when administering vaccines

2. Check and record client information accurately including permission to use mobile numbers for text alerts

3. Confirm client's identity (Name, address, date of birth and mother or father's name as appropriate. For younger children it will be necessary to confirm identity with parent/legal guardian)

4. Provides appropriate information regarding the vaccines to be administered including the risk of vaccinating and not vaccinating

5. Obtains written informed consent

6. Assesses the client's suitability for immunisation on the day. Vaccines should be given to clients for whom no contraindication is identified as per the Immunisation Guidelines of Ireland

7. Routine physical examinations and procedures (e.g. measuring temperatures) are NOT recommended for vaccinating persons who appear to be healthy. The client or parent should be asked if the person being vaccinated is ill

8. Defer any clients with an acute febrile illness on the day and reschedules vaccination

9. Ensure that when vaccines are being given according to a particular schedule e.g. PCIP that the interval from last vaccines given is appropriate. If not, vaccination should be deferred and the client rescheduled

10. Check that the intervals between different vaccines are appropriate

11. Check that the vaccine has been prescribed by the GP or that the vaccine can be administered under medicine protocol

12. Check that the appropriate vaccine(s) are in the vaccine fridge, are in date and stored in accordance with cold chain directions

13. Remove vaccine from the vaccine fridge when the client is ready for vaccination

14. Verify with the parent/legal guardian/client or other health professional that the correct vaccine is being given, the expiry date has not passed and records this on the form

15. Wash hands or uses disinfectant gel using correct techniques before vaccine administration

16. Reconstitute vaccines in accordance with manufacturer's instruction

References
Refer to main HSE Immunisation Guidelines and HSE (2018). Guidelines for vaccination in General Practice. HSE National Immunisation Office: Dublin

88. Guidelines for Administering IM Vaccines

This route is used for the majority of vaccines

Age Months	Site	Needle Size mm	gauge
Birth to 12 months*	Anterolateral aspect of middle or upper thigh	25	23-25
12 to 36	Anterolateral aspect of middle or upper thigh until deltoid has developed adequate muscle mass	25	23-25
From 3 years onwards**	Most dense portion of the deltoid muscle– between acromion and muscle insertion	25	23-25
*: Use a 16mm length needle in infants under 2.5-3kgs; **: Use 40mm length needle on women>90kgs, men >118kgs			

1. It is not necessary to use gloves for routine intradermal, subcutaneous and intramuscular injections, unless likely to come into contact with potentially infectious body fluids or unless the health care worker has a lesion on his or her hand

2. If gloves are worn they should be changed for each patient. If the skin at the injection site is visibly dirty it should be cleaned with soap and water

3. There is no need to use a disinfectant e.g. alcohol swabs. If an alcohol swab is used, injection should be delayed for 30 seconds to ensure the alcohol will have evaporated

4. Spread the skin of the administration site taut between the thumb and forefinger (to avoid injecting into subcutaneous tissue and to isolate the muscle)

5. In small infants and others with little muscle mass the tissue around the injection site may be gently bunched up

6. Insert the needle rapidly and fully at a 90 degree angle to the skin. Inject the vaccine into the muscle over 1-2 seconds

7. Rapidly withdraw the needle and apply light pressure to the injection site for several seconds with a dry cotton ball or gauze

8. Multiple injections given in the same limb should be separated by at least 2.5 cm

89. Administering Vaccines by Subcutaneous Injection

Use this route for yellow fever vaccine. May also be used for varicella and MMR vaccines and in those with severe bleeding disorders. There are only two routinely recommended SC sites for administration of vaccines, the middle third of the anterolateral thigh and the deltoid region (upper arm)

Procedure

1. Insert needle at 45 degree angle to the skin
2. Gently pinch up SC tissue to prevent injecting into muscle
3. There is no need to aspirate prior to injection as there are no large blood vessels at the preferred injection sites
4. Multiple injections given in the same limb should be separated by at least 2.5cm

90. Administering Vaccines by Oral Route

Oral typhoid vaccine

The capsule should be taken approximately one hour before a meal with a cold or lukewarm drink. The vaccine capsule should not be chewed and should be swallowed as soon as possible after placing in the mouth.

Rotavirus vaccines Rotarix (RV1):

Remove the protective tip cap from the applicator. The child should be seated in a reclining position. Administer the entire contents of the vaccine applicator into the child's mouth, towards the inner cheek.

Rotateq (RV5)

Tear open the pouch and remove the dosing tube. Clear the fluid from the dispensing tip by holding tube vertically and tapping cap. Puncture the dispensing tip by screwing cap clockwise until it becomes tight. Administer dose by gently squeezing liquid into infant's mouth until dosing tube is empty. (A residual drop may remain in the tip of the tube)

Post Administration of Vaccine

1. Dispose of sharps immediately, without recapping the needle, into the sharps containers provided. Discard the empty oral applicator and tip cap into approved biological waste containers

2. Wash hands or uses disinfectant gel according to correct techniques

3. Complete the administration details including the vaccine name, manufacturer, batch number and expiry date, using peel off labels provided where appropriate, at the end of the consent form immediately after the vaccine is given. For reconstituted vaccines the batch number recorded is the one on the box and on the peel off labels

References
Refer to main HSE Immunisation Guidelines and HSE (2018). Guidelines for vaccination in General Practice. HSE National Immunisation Office: Dublin

Useful Websites and Links to Health Services

General Health Websites

https://www.hse.ie/eng/

https://www.hse.ie/eng/services/list/

http://www.irishhealth.com/

https://patient.info/health

http://undertheweather.ie/

Contraception and STI Information Websites

http://www.thinkcontraception.ie/

https://spunout.ie/health/article/sti-clinics-ireland

http://www.irishhealth.com/clin/sexual_health/index.html

Mental Health Website

http://www.yourmentalhealth.ie/

https://www.hse.ie/eng/services/list/4/mental-health-services/

http://www.mentalhealthireland.ie

http://www.aware.ie

Alcohol and Drug related Websites

http://www.askaboutalcohol.ie/

https://www.hse.ie/eng/health/hl/change/alcohol/

http://www.drinkaware.ie/facts/alcohol-in-ireland

http://www.drugs.ie/phone

Screening Services Information Website

https://www.screeningservice.ie/

Immunisation Information Websites

https://www.hse.ie/eng/health/immunisation/

https://www.hse.ie/eng/health/child/meningitis/

Travel Vaccination Information Websites

https://www.hse.ie/eng/health/az/t/travel-vaccinations/

https://www.hse.ie/eng/health/immunisation/pubinfo/adult/travelvacc/

Nutrition/ Healthy Eating Website

https://spunout.ie/health/category/healthy-eating

https://www.hse.ie/healthyeating

https://www.hse.ie/eng/about/who/healthwellbeing/our-priority- programmes/heal/healthy-eating-guidelines/

Medicines Information Online

http://www.medicines.ie

Quick links to Common Conditions

Home/Self Care Advice and Treatments

Cold: http://undertheweather.ie/ailment/cold

Flu: http://undertheweather.ie/ailment/flu

Cough: http://undertheweather.ie/ailment/cough

Sore Throat: http://undertheweather.ie/ailment/throat

Earache: http://undertheweather.ie/ailment/ear

Rash: http://undertheweather.ie/ailment/rash

Fever: http://undertheweather.ie/ailment/temperature

Vomiting: http://undertheweather.ie/ailment/tummy

References

- An Bord Altranais (2000). Scope of Nursing and Midwifery Practice Framework. ABA: Dublin.

- An Bord Altranais (2000). The Code of Professional Conduct for each Nurse and Midwife. ABA: Dublin.

- An Bord Altranais (2002). Recording Clinical Practice: Guidance to Nurses and Midwives on the Development of Policies, Guidelines and Protocols. ABA: Dublin.

- An Bord Altranais (2007). Guidance to Nurses and Midwives on Medication Management. ABA: Dublin.

- AHA (2015). Guideline Updates for CPR and ECC. American Heart Association: USA.

- Baumann, J.J (2009). *Neurologic clinical assessment and diagnostic procedures.* In Urden, L.Stacey, K. & Logh, M. (eds) Critical Care Nursing: Diagnosis and Management, 6th edn. St Louis: MO: Mosby, pp. 700-723.

- Bickley, L. Szilagyi, P. Hoffman, R. (2009). *Bates Guide to Physical Examination and History Taking.* 10th edn. Philadelphia: Lipincott Williams & Wilkins.

- Bickley, L. Szilagyi, P. Hoffman, R. (2017). *Bates Guide to Physical Examination and History Taking.* 12th edn. Philadelphia: Lipincott Williams & Wilkins.

- Bravery, K. (1999). Paediatric Intravenous Therapy in Children. In Dougherty, L. and Lambe, J. Intravenous Therapy in Nursing Practice. Churchill Livingston: London.

- British Society for Clinical Cytology (2003). Taking Cervical Smears. BSCC: London.

- Bruns TB and Worthington JM (2000). Using tissue adhesive for wound repair: a practical guide to dermabond. American Family Physician 61(5):1383-1388.

- Cervical Check (2011). Guide for smear takers 2nd Edition. The National Cancer Screening Service: Ireland.

- Cheshire Ireland (2013). Standard Procedure for the Irrigating (flushing) of an Indwelling Catheter, Document Number: CLSP 29, Version Number: 2, Version Date: 31/05/2013. Cheshire Ireland.

- Cole, E., Lynch, A., Reynolds, T, (2008). Wound care. In Dolan B and Holt L (eds) Accident and Emergency: Theory into Practice, 2nd edition. Balliere Tindall: London.

- Department of Health and Children (2012). A Strategic Framework for Reform of the Health Service 2012– 2015 available at www.dohc.ie/publications

- Department of Health and Children (2015). Management of an Acute Asthma Attack in Adults (aged 16 years and older) National Clinical Guideline No. 14. An Roinn Slainte DOH: Dublin.

- Department of Health and Children (2016). Irish College of General Practitioners. A Practical Guide to Integrated Type 2 Diabetes Care. DOH: Dublin.

- Department of Health and Children (2018). Adult type 1 diabetes mellitus (NCEC National Clinical Guideline No. 17). DOH: Dublin.

- Dougherty, L. (2008). Peripheral Cannulation. Nursing Standard. 22 (52), 49-56.

- Dougherty, L. & Lister, S. (2009). The Royal Marsden Hospital Manual of Clinical Nursing Procedures. 7th Ed. Wiley Blackwell Pub: Chichester.

- Dougherty, L. & Lister, S. (2015). The Royal Marsden Hospital Manual of Clinical Nursing Procedures. 9th Ed. Wiley Blackwell Pub: Chichester.

- Ellingson K, Haas JP, Aiello AE, Kusek L, Maragakis LL, Olmsted RN *et al.* (2014). Strategies to prevent healthcare-associated infections through hand hygiene. *Infect Control Hosp Epidemiol*; 35(8):937-60.

- Farion KJ, Russell KF, Osmond MH, Hartling L, Klassen TP, Durec T, Vandermeer B (2009). Tissue adhesives for traumatic lacerations in children and adults (Cochrane Review). The Cochrane Library. Issue 1, Chichester UK: John Willey and Sons Ltd.

- Fuller, G. (2008). *Neurological Examination Made Easy*, 4TH edn. Edinburgh: Churchill Livingstone.

- Health Protection and Surveillance Centre (2009). Prevention of Intravascular Catheter Related Infection in Ireland. HPSC: Dublin

- Health Protection and Surveillance Centre (2009). Peripheral Vascular Catheter Care Bundle HPSC: Dublin. Health Information and Quality Authority (2015). Medicines Management Guidance. HIQA: Dublin.

- Hinds, P., Quargnenti, A., Gattuso, J., Srivastava, D. (2002). Comparing the results of coagulation tests on blood drawn by venepuncture and through heparinised tunnelled venous access devices in patients with cancer. Oncology Nursing Forum; 29(3) E26-E34.

- Hollander JE, Singer AJ. (1999). Laceration management. Annals of Emergency Medicine 34(3):356-67.

- Health Service Executive (2007). Guidelines for Nursing and Midwifery Staff Undertaking Adult Peripheral Venepuncture. HSE: Dublin.

- Health Service Executive (2008). A Practical Guide to Immunisations. HSE: Dublin.

- Health Service Executive (2010). A Guiding Framework for Education, Training and Competence Validation in Venepuncture and Peripheral Intravenous Cannulation for Nurses and Midwives. HSE: Dublin.

- Health Service Executive (2010). National Clinical Policy and Procedural Guidelines for Nurses and Midwives undertaking Peripheral Cannulation in Adults. HSE: Dublin.

- Health Service Executive (2010). Guidelines for the Care and Maintenance of Long Term Central Venous Access Devices (CVAD's) in University Hospital Waterford excluding Dialysis Lines. UHW: Waterford.

- Health Service Executive (2010). Healthcare Risk Waste Management Segregation Packaging and Storage Guidelines for healthcare Risk Waste. HSE: Dublin.

- Health Service Executive (2011). Policy for the Administration of Intravenous Medicinal Preparations by Nursing and Midwifery Staff. HSE: Dublin.

- Health Service Executive (2012). Guidelines for the administration of medications. HSE: Dublin.

- Health Service Executive (2012). Guidelines for the administration of subcutaneous medications. HSE: Dublin.

- Health Service Executive (2012). Guidelines for Nursing and Midwifery Staff undertaking adult Intravenous Cannulation. HSE: Dublin.

- Health Service Executive (2012). Brief Intervention for Smoking Cessation National Training Programme. Participant Resource. HSE: Dublin.

- Health Service Executive (2013). National Policy for the Administration of Intravenous Medication by Registered Nurses and Midwives. HSE: Dublin.

- Health Service Executive (2015). Royal College of Physicians Ireland. Guidelines for hand hygiene in Irish healthcare settings. HSE: Ireland.

- Health Service Executive (2016). Directions for Nurses and Midwives for the Management of a Patient who Develops Anaphylaxis and Medicine Protocol for the Administration of Epinephrine (Adrenaline) Injection BP 1: 1,000 by IM Injection by Registered Nurses and Midwives. HSE: Dublin.

- Health Service Executive (2017). Clinical Competence in Male Adult Urethral Catheterisation. Continence Promotion Unit. Dr Steeven's Hospital. HSE: Dublin.

- Health Service Executive (2017). Clinical Competence in Female Catheterisation. Continence Promotion Unit. Dr Steeven's Hospital. HSE: Dublin.

- Health Service Executive (2017). Clinical Competence in Suprapubic Re-catheterisation. Continence Promotion Unit. Dr Steeven's Hospital. HSE: Dublin.

- Health Service Executive (2018). Primary Childhood Immunisation Schedule. HSE: Dublin.

- Health Service Executive (2018). School Programme Immunisations Schedule. HSE: Dublin.

- Health Service Executive (2018). Guidelines for vaccination in General Practice. HSE National Immunisation Office: Dublin.

- Health Service Executive (2018). Acute Hospital Laboratory Supplies. Type of Specimen Containers. HSE: Dublin.

- Irish College of General Practitioners (2017). HSE/ICGP Weight Management Treatment Algorithm for Adults. ICGP: Dublin.

- Irish College of General Practitioners (2017). BMI Chart for use with the Weight Management Treatment Algorithm for Adults. ICGP: Dublin.

- Loveday, H. Wilson, J. Pratt, R. Golsorki, M. Tingle, A. Bak, A. et al. epic3 (2014). National Evidence-Based Guidelines for Preventing Healthcare-Associated Infections in NHS Hospitals in England. J Hosp Inf.;86 Suppl 1:S1-70.

- Mayo, D.J., Dimond, E.P., Kramer, W., McDonald, K.H. (1996). Discard volumes necessary for clinically useful coagulation studies from heparinised Hickman catheters. Oncology Nursing Forum; 23 (4):671-675.

- Medical Council (2009). Guide to professional conduct and ethics for registered medical practitioners, 7th Edition. Dublin.

- National Health Service (2010). Guidelines for the Care and Maintenance of Central Venous Access Devices. Sutton and Merton NHS Trust: England.

- National Institute for Health and Care Excellence (2012). Infection: prevention and control of healthcare- associated infections in primary and community care. Partial update of NICE Clinical Guideline 2. National Clinical Guideline Centre: UK.

- National Institute for Health and Care Excellence (2014). 'Head injury', NICE clinical guideline 176. NICE: UK.

- Nursing and Midwifery Board of Ireland (2014). Code of Professional Conduct and Ethics for Registered Nurses and Registered Midwives. NMBI: Dublin.

- Nursing and Midwifery Board of Ireland (2015). Scope of Nursing and Midwifery Practice Framework for Registered Nurses and Registered Midwives. NMBI: Dublin.

- Nursing and Midwifery Board of Ireland (2015). Ethical Conduct in Research: Professional guidance. NMBI: Dublin.

- Nursing and Midwifery Board of Ireland (2015). Quality Clinical Learning Environment: Professional guidance. NMBI: Dublin.

- Nursing and Midwifery Board of Ireland (2015). Recording Clinical Practice: Professional guidance. NMBI: Dublin.

- Nursing and Midwifery Board of Ireland (2015). Working with Older People: Professional guidance. NMBI: Dublin.

- Nursing and Midwifery Board of Ireland (2018). Practice Standards and Guidelines for Nurses and Midwives with Prescriptive Authority (3rd Edition). NMBI: Dublin.

- Our Lady's Children's Hospital, Crumlin (2012). Nursing Practice Committee Guidelines on the Use of Tissue Adhesive for Minor Laceration Repair. OLCHC: Dublin.

- Philips, P. (2000). Issues Relating to the Use of Disposable and Reusable Speculum. Surgical Material Testing Laboratory: UK.

- Pratt. R., J., Pellowe. C., M., and Wilson. J. A., (2007). EPIC 2: National Evidence-Based Guidelines for Preventing Healthcare-Associated Infections in NHS Hospitals in England. The Journal of Hospital Infection 655, 51-564.

- Prochaska, J.O. & DiClemente, C.C (1982). 'Trans-theoretical Therapy: Towards a More Integrative Model of Change' Psychotherapy: Research, Theory & Practice 19(3) pp.276-288.

- Prochaska, J.O., DiClemente, C.C & Norcross, J.C. (1992). 'In Search of How People Change: Applications to Addictive Behaviours' American Psychologist 47 (9) pp.1102-1114.

- Provincial Infectious Diseases Advisory Committee (2014). Best Practices for Hand Hygiene in all Health Care Settings, 4th edition. Public Health Ontario.

- Quality in Practice Committee (2012). Asthma control in General Practice 2nd ed. Adapted from the GINA Global Strategy for Asthma Management and Prevention. Ireland.

- Rosenthal, J., Rymer, J., Jones, R., Haldane, S., Cohen, S., Bartholomew, J. (2005). Chaperones for Intimate Examinations: Cross Sectional Survey of Attitudes and Practices of General Practitioners. BMJ 2005; 330; 234-235

- Royal Collage of Nursing (2008). Catheter Care Guidance for Nurses. RCN: London. Royal Collage of Nursing (2012). Catheter Care Guidance for Nurses. RCN: London.

- Royal Collage of Nursing (2014). Competencies: An Education and Training Competence Framework for Peripheral Venous Cannulation in Children and Young People: RCN: London.

- Royal Collage of Nursing (2017). Guidelines for the administration of medications. RCN: London.

- Royal Collage of Nursing (2017). Guidelines for the administration of subcutaneous anticoagulant medications. RCN: London.

- SARI Infection Control Subcommittee (2012). Guidelines for Hand Hygiene in the Irish Health Care Settings. Health Protection Surveillance Centre. Ireland.

- Scales, K. (2005). Vascular Access: A Guide to Peripheral Venous Cannulation. Nursing Standard. 19 (49) pp. 48-52.

- Society for Cardiological Science and Technology (2014). Clinical Guidelines by Consensus. Recording a Standard 12 Lead Electrocardiogram. SCST: UK.

- St Luke's Hospital (2011). Policy for the Administration of Intravenous Medicinal Preparations by Nursing and Midwifery Staff; St Luke's Hospital. Kilkenny, Ireland.

- St Luke's Hospital (2011). Guidelines for Enteral Feeding, St Luke's Hospital, Kilkenny, Ireland.

- St Luke's Hospital (2013). Policies and Procedures: Emergency Gastrostomy Replacement with Balloon Tube. St Luke's Hospital. Kilkenny, Ireland.

- St Luke's Hospital (2013). Policies and Procedures: Revised Guidelines for Enteral Feeding. Inserting Corflo Replacement Gastrostomy tubes, St Luke's Hospital. Kilkenny, Ireland.

- St Luke's Hospital (2013). Policies and Procedures: Revised Guidelines for Enteral Feeding. Inserting Corflo Replacement Gastrostomy tubes. Document Reference No: SLGH DTN 001 Revision No: 1 Approval Date: Nov 2013. St Luke's Hospital. Kilkenny, Ireland.

- St Luke's Hospital (2013). Policies and Procedures: Revised Guidelines for Enteral Feeding (2013) Inserting Corflo Replacement Cubby Gastrostomy tubes. Document Reference No: SLGH DTN 001 Revision No: 1 Approval Date: Nov 2013. St Luke's Hospital. Kilkenny, Ireland.

- University Health Network (2010). Clinical Policies: Vascular Access - Port Site Access, Care and Maintenance, USA.

- University Hospital Waterford (2018). Guidelines for the Care and Maintenance of Long Term Central Venous Access Devices (CVAD's). UHW. Waterford

- World Health Organisation (2009). Guidelines on Hand Hygiene in Health Care. WHO: Geneva.

- World Health Organisation (2012). Hand hygiene in outpatient and home-based care and long-term care facilities. WHO: Geneva.

Images

Authors own or sourced via creative commons.org at: https://search.creativecommons.org/

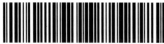
27430022R00132

Printed in Great Britain
by Amazon